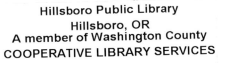

This Narrow Space

This Narrow Space

A PEDIATRIC ONCOLOGIST,
HIS JEWISH, MUSLIM,
AND CHRISTIAN PATIENTS, AND
A HOSPITAL IN JERUSALEM

Elisha Waldman

SCHOCKEN BOOKS, NEW YORK

Copyright © 2018 by Elisha Waldman

All rights reserved. Published in the United States by Schocken Books, a division of Penguin Random House LLC, New York, and distributed in Canada by Random House of Canada, a division of Penguin Random House Canada Limited, Toronto.

Schocken Books and colophon are registered trademarks of Penguin Random House LLC.

Grateful acknowledgment is made to Farrar, Straus and Giroux for permission to reprint an excerpt of "Try to Remember Some Details" from The Poetry of Yehuda Amichai by Yehuda Amichai, edited by Robert Alter. Copyright © 2015 by Hana Amichai. Introduction and selection copyright © 2015 by Robert Alter. Reprinted by permission of Farrar, Straus and Giroux.

A portion of this work first appeared, in different form, in Bellevue Literary Review, vol. 14, no. 1 (Spring 2014).

Library of Congress Cataloging-in-Publication Data
Name: Waldman, Elisha, author.
Title: This narrow space : a pediatric oncologist, his Jewish, Muslim, and Christian patients, and a hospital in Jerusalem / Elisha Waldman.
Description: First edition. New York : Schocken, 2018
Identifiers: LCCN 2017031186. ISBN 9780805243321 (hardback).
ISBN 9780805243338 (ebook). ISBN 9780805212754 (open market).
Subjects: LCSH: Waldman, Elisha. Oncologists—Jerusalem—Biography.
Cancer in children—Social aspects—Jerusalem. Bet ha-òholim
"Hadasah" (Jerusalem)—Employees—Biography. BISAC: BIOGRAPHY &
AUTOBIOGRAPHY/Medical. MEDICAL/Pediatric Emergencies.
Classification: LCC RC265.8.W35 A3 2018. DDC 616.99/40092 [B] — dc23.
LC record available at lccn.loc.gov/2017031186

www.schocken.com

Jacket images: (door) adrian 825 / Getty Images;
(bed) Blend Images / Getty Images
Jacket design by Oliver Munday
Book design by Iris Weinstein

Printed in the United States of America
First Edition
2 4 6 8 9 7 5 3 1

For Sasha and Lev,
who broadened my horizons beyond my dreams

TRY TO REMEMBER SOME DETAILS

Try to remember some details.
Remember the clothing
of the one you love
so that on the day of loss you'll be able to say: last seen
wearing such-and-such, brown jacket, white hat.

Try to remember some details.

For they have no face
and their soul is hidden and their crying
is the same as their laughter,
and their silence and their shouting rise to one height
and their body temperature is between 98 and 104 degrees
and they have no life outside this narrow space
and they have no graven image, no likeness, no memory
and they have paper cups on the day of their rejoicing
and paper cups that are used once only.

Try to remember some details.

For the world
is filled with people who were torn from their sleep
with no one to mend the tear,
and unlike wild beasts they live
each in his lonely hiding place and they die
together on battlefields
and in hospitals.

And the earth will swallow all of them,
good and evil together, like the followers of Korah,
all of them in their rebellion against death,
their mouths open till the last moment,
praising and cursing in a single
howl.

Try, try
to remember some details.

—YEHUDA AMICHAI

This Narrow Space

1

Protocols

I'M SURE I'VE BEEN HERE BEFORE, but I can't remember exactly when. Perhaps when I was younger, on one of our summer vacations in Israel, hiking in the cool forest or exploring one of the ancient churches in the village. But maybe I'm just imagining it, willing the feeling into existence. All I know, as I drive down into the valley of Ein Kerem in Jerusalem, is that everything here feels familiar. And when I walk through the doors of the Department of Pediatric Hematology-Oncology at Hadassah Hospital, it feels as though I'm arriving at a place that I know from my dreams.

As I make my way down the corridor, the first thing I see is two boys, no more than four years old, sitting alongside each other, playing at a low table in the waiting area. In one poignant snapshot they capture all of my Zionist ideals. They would be indistinguishable from any other kids their age except for the fact that they both have the shiny, immaculately bald scalps that are the unmistakable by-products of chemotherapy treatments.

Oblivious to the dull hospital decor, the lifeless fluorescent illumination, the bustle that surrounds them, the pain and the drama that are endemic to a place like this, the boys work side by side with brightly colored construction paper and crayons. One, whose *kippah* has slipped off his head and lies upended on the table, is obviously Jewish. He's hunched over his project, focusing so intently on collaborating with the little boy next to him that he doesn't even notice his *kippah* has come off. The other boy, closely attended by a woman in a long *abaya* and *hijab,* is clearly Muslim. The boys play together, sharing crayons and comparing creations as though nothing, not religion, not cancer, not politics or war, could get in the way. For a liberal American Jewish pediatric oncologist at the start of his career it's the Zionist dream come true, and it's for this that I've made aliyah, moving to Israel from the United States. It's March of 2007, it's my first day on the job, and I'm eager to begin. I hurry past the boys, on my way to meet with my first patient.

Though unhappy families may indeed be unhappy in their own way, my experience has been that when it comes to children facing life-threatening illness, unhappy families often actually have a great deal in common. I am relying on this theory for guidance as I begin my new job as attending physician at Hadassah, hoping to translate my experience in the United States into practice here in Israel. Despite the obvious cultural differences, I figure the common language of illness will provide a bridge to ease me into my new environment.

On this first day of work I am still awash in the exuberance and sense of limitless possibility that is typical of comfortably situated expats who have made aliyah. As my patient and her parents walk into the exam room, before even a word is exchanged, I recognize the familiar tension from so many similar situations I'd experienced in New York. I glance down at my patient's chart. Lena, a seventeen-year-old Israeli Arab, has been having increasing pain in her left leg over the past two months.

A recent X-ray showed what looked like a mass, and a biopsy has now determined that Lena has osteosarcoma, a malignant tumor of bone. There is no evidence that the tumor has spread elsewhere, so her prognosis is relatively good, about a 70 percent chance of long-term survival. But the treatment will be far from simple, and the outcome far from certain. Lena and her parents have come here today to hear the results of all the recent testing. They have undoubtedly gathered hints from previous meetings with my colleagues that this may turn out to be cancer. After all, they have come to a place called "Department of Pediatric Hematology-Oncology." But I know they are hoping, until the very moment that I give them the diagnosis, that this will all turn out to be a horrible mistake.

My role at Hadassah is to oversee the care of children with sarcomas, which are any one of a myriad number of solid tumors that form in such areas as the bone, muscle, and connective tissue. Because this is my first day and I am still getting oriented, I will be joined by the director of the department, Dr. Mickey Weintraub, who already met with Lena and her parents at her initial referral. I'm grateful for his presence. Although I have spent a great deal of my pre-aliyah life in Israel (I even attended medical school in Tel Aviv) and there is much that should be familiar to me, the way these initial conversations are carried out is so important in shaping the ongoing relationship between oncologist and patient, so critical in setting the stage for how decisions will be made, that I am wary of diving in by myself on my first day. I have, over the past few years, done this many times in the United States, first as a trainee and then for a year and a half as an attending physician. But I find myself worrying about the language barrier, the cultural nuances, the way in which I should be both delivering information and responding to cues from this young woman and her family. The intimacy of these discussions can be intense, and though this intimacy can be deeply rewarding, it can also be intimidating. I have taken up residence in Israel feeling fairly linguistically and culturally competent, able to manage the activities of daily living, but telling a seventeen-year-old Israeli Arab that she has a life-threatening condition is a very different challenge. In many ways, I feel I am starting my training all over again.

When Lena and her parents arrive, I am still preparing the office for the meeting: organizing chairs, getting the clutter out of the way, making sure there are tissues on the desk, unobtrusive but handy, available for the tears that will surely come. As they enter, I try to compensate for the language barrier by smiling and giving them a hearty "shalom." I come around from behind the desk and stick my hand out in greeting. Lena, limping, lags behind, so her mother is the first person to whom I offer my hand. She stares at it awkwardly, and everyone stops, unsure what to do. It takes a moment for me to register that both she and her daughter are wearing *hijabs,* and that for them physical contact with any man other than immediate family members is prohibited. Lena's father kindly rescues us, dodging around his wife and thrusting his hand into mine, pumping it firmly while Lena and her mother slide into their seats. I retreat behind the desk. I am already worried that I have just compounded this family's anxiety by introducing an element of cultural discomfort. I realize how much I'm worrying, and I worry even more that they can sense this.

Mickey and the Arabic-speaking social worker have not yet arrived, leaving us all drowning together in a tense, painful silence. My Arabic is barely good enough at this point to say good morning, let alone to make small talk to try to put them at ease, and Lena's parents speak virtually no Hebrew. Perhaps it's better that way: they can't start asking me difficult questions while I am feeling new, alone, and exposed. I pointlessly tidy the desktop while we all smile uncomfortably at one another. I mostly try to avoid making eye contact with Lena's parents, though I can feel their eyes probing my face, my body language, for some hint as to what is coming. Lena is slouched down in her seat. She's a lanky teenager, with her hair modestly covered in a plain blue headscarf. She is also wearing a rhinestone-studded sweatshirt, blue jeans, and sneakers. It's a curious and charming blend of Western teenage fashion and Middle Eastern religious sensibility. Sparkles of glitter on her sneakers remind me that though we are about to have a very adult conversation, this young woman is still in many ways a child. She stares at the floor. I sense she must know in her heart what she is about to hear.

I take some comfort in the elements here that are familiar, mentally breaking the situation down into its fundamental components and reviewing the steps we are about to take. In oncology training we learn the concept of the "day-one talk," the essential elements that a clinician must cover in order to start moving forward with treatment. These include explaining what cancer is, why it is so dangerous, and what type of cancer the patient has. We also discuss treatments and their side effects and risks. And somewhere in there, though we focus on hope, we bring up the possibility of death. Lena's thin, bony arms, evident under the loose sleeves of her hoodie, as well as her slightly sunken cheeks tell me that she is already suffering the metabolic effects of having a large and growing tumor in her body. This is the paradox of cancer: exuberantly unrestrained cells keep dividing with no respect for boundaries or pacing, no ear for the rhythm of life, and this is what leads to death.

Once we have navigated the day-one talk, there are procedures that will have to be scheduled before treatment can begin. There will be an echocardiogram to make sure Lena's cardiac muscle can handle the chemotherapy and to establish a baseline to monitor for future damage, a hearing test (for similar reasons), and perhaps the removal and freezing of an ovary to mitigate the infertility that will almost certainly result from the chemo. We will need to reserve an operating room for the insertion of a port under the skin of Lena's chest—a silicon bubble attached to a small tube that feeds into a deep blood vessel. Inserting a needle through the skin and into the bubble with each course of chemotherapy will lessen the possibility of infection and allow for safer administration of our toxic medications.

Reviewing these elements calms me—my own Buddhist-like mantra. There is a moment of quiet just before the discussion with the patient begins, similar to what I imagine goes on backstage at a performance as the actors take their places before the curtain rises. I experience it as though time has slowed, and I wonder if the patients and their families experience the same thing, these last few moments when they can hope that this will all just go away. It's a time when even I sometimes fantasize that this is simply a bad dream from which I can awake and the child will be fine. I use this time to clear my thoughts, to say a quiet prayer—to any god that may be listening—for wisdom and clarity in what we are about to do.

As if sensing my readiness, Mickey and the social worker finally arrive, and we can begin. A native-born Israeli Jew, Mickey is a kind and unassuming man. He leads by example, rarely resorts to discipline, and is deeply loved by staff and patients alike. A full three years before making aliyah I met him while on a job-scouting visit to Israel and knew within minutes that someday I would end up working for this man. I find myself addressing him as "boss" or "sir" as a half-joking sign of respect. He would never expect anyone to treat him with such formality, though he very much deserves it. He's omnipresent in the department, and I will come to appreciate how much his calm demeanor contributes to the safe space that this place represents.

The social worker is a young Israeli Arab woman who is here as much to lend support to Lena and her family as to act as a translator and cultural mediator for us. Mickey begins gently but with purpose, and the discussion proceeds rapidly. He moves deftly, like an experienced surgeon neatly dissecting layer after layer of tissue to expose an injured organ, following a template that I am more or less familiar with from the United States. It again strikes me that there are elements of this work that are universal. Regardless of nationality, ethnicity, or religion, the goals and challenges of the day-one talk are pretty basic. In this first meeting the family will likely absorb only a limited amount of the information presented. Give them what they need to begin the process, but recognize that, as treatment progresses, there will have to be many more discussions to reinforce what we are attempting to convey and to elaborate on it as necessary.

The conversation takes on its own rhythm, in part because of the need for translation. I have worked through interpreters in the past, but perhaps because I'm full of adrenaline, at this moment I am particularly aware of this rhythm. Mickey and I speak English with each other, conferring about what information to present next or how to respond to a question. He then conveys our response in Hebrew to the social worker, who in turn translates it into Arabic for Lena and her parents. They respond in Arabic, which is translated back to Hebrew by the social worker, and Mickey then translates it into English for me to make sure I understand. The whole process, while in some respects cumbersome, takes on an ebb-and-flow that provides, at least for me, a certain comfort. The pauses allow me time to think, to evaluate their responses, to watch their body language, and to think about where we should next steer the conversation. I know from past experience that these discussions can easily devolve into fear, anger, or even outright panic. But now, the very regularity of the conversational rhythm gives the room a sense of order and control that I, and hopefully the family, find reassuring.

Lena does not speak. Her mother, wide-eyed, lips trembling, fingers working a tear-soaked tissue to shreds, radiates waves of desperation as she speaks—no translation is necessary. Lena's father, buttoned-down, expressionless, asks just one or two concrete, pragmatic questions: prognosis, next steps. They return again and again to the leg and the question of amputation. We assure them that almost all tumors like Lena's can be removed with limb-sparing surgery, but we also slip in that we can't make any promises, that it is a surgical decision, and that it depends in part on how the tumor responds to the chemotherapy. In short, that we hope but we don't know for certain. Typically, patients with this sort of tumor start off with about three months of chemotherapy, both to shrink the tumor and to mop up any cancerous cells that may have already escaped and spread, in numbers too low to detect, to other parts of the body. We hope that amputation will not be necessary, but starting cancer therapy is something of an act of faith, with many unknowns down the road.

The meeting draws to a close. There is only so long a patient and her family can be subjected to this sort of conversation, and we want to allow them time to process what they have been told, to formulate new questions, and to begin to adjust to their new reality.

And we, too, must move on. Despite the intimacy of these meetings, they are often just one in a series of many similar interactions throughout the day, and we have to be mindful of the need to allow other children to be seen, to give other parents the opportunity to ask questions. It almost feels deceitful the way we carefully orchestrate these interactions, so full of emotion, only to repeat the scene moments later in another room but with a different set of players. It's not that the emotions are false, the empathy we convey fabricated, but there is something manufactured about the way in which we are genuinely present in each discussion while still managing to create some emotional space within ourselves for the next one. It's a skill, though not one you're ever taught. And it's certainly a skill that, if not done well, runs risks, either of clinician burnout or of projecting insincerity to patients. But I'm young and I'm still trying to figure this all out, to understand where to put all this baggage as the day races on from patient to patient.

In wrapping up with Lena's family we emphasize the positive, stressing the fact that most children with this type of tumor survive. We focus on the next steps. We present them with a printed-out description of the treatment protocol, a standardized map of all planned treatments, which in Lena's case is specific for the management of osteosarcoma. The protocol outlines day by day and week by week all the specifics of treatment, including what type of chemotherapy will be given, routes of administration, doses, rates, and various possible adjustments. It shows us when to pause, when to reevaluate, when to stop, and when to consider a different approach. Of course, it doesn't capture the innumerable elements we can't foresee and that are so much harder to quantify, such as the side effects—the nausea, the weakness, the fevers and infections—and, of course, the dreaded cancer recurrences. Though they may appear frightening, even overwhelming at first, especially as families assess line after line of difficult treatments, at the same time these protocols, each tailored for a different type of cancer, outline a path to a cure, and therefore may provide a measure of comfort. Just as the rhythm of the translated conversation comforted me despite the element of fear and danger in the room, so a treatment protocol may, in its regularity and predictability, impart to families and clinicians alike a sense of safety and control. Protocols give us at least some sense of what to expect, to see what is coming. They allow us to impose some sort of order on a life that has been thrown into chaos and uncertainty. Rabbi Abraham Joshua Heschel, one of the great Jewish thinkers of the twentieth century, writes about the "architecture of time." He discusses the idea specifically in the context of ritual and the religious calendar, suggesting that if we don't know where things begin and end, we can't possibly know where we are now, resulting in a distressing and even destructive inability to locate ourselves in space and time. Religious ritual and the sacred calendar help create this architecture of time, forging a structure of safe space and rhythm in an otherwise chaotic and unpredictable world. Pediatric oncology treatment protocols work the same way: they become sacred calendars, a set of rituals allowing us, in the face of danger and uncertainty, to locate ourselves, giving us a sense of how we might safely navigate what lies ahead. As we present Lena and her parents with the protocol, our intention is for them to find comfort in having a plan, in knowing that there is a clearly delineated timeline and set of rituals that will ultimately carry them safely to the end.

Before they leave, we also lay out a more immediate plan for the next few days, before the chemotherapy begins. The social worker plans to follow up the next day by phone, and in two days Lena will return to complete her pretreatment tests. We say our farewells and, despite the nature of the meeting, I feel encouraged. Though of course my heart goes out to Lena, this is exactly why I came to Israel: for the opportunity to navigate the new languages, the blend of cultures, the political complexity. This family is at once foreign and familiar to me, a piece of the beautiful cultural jigsaw puzzle that is Israel. Lena's family is ethnically Palestinian Arab, but they live just outside of Jerusalem, within the city's municipal boundaries, and are therefore Israeli citizens. They are Muslims living in a predominantly Jewish, Western society. Despite my earlier anxiety, I am already looking forward to our next meeting, to engaging more deeply with them. As a newly minted Israeli, I am here not just as an observer, not as a tourist, but as someone participating in and actively engaging with society in a meaningful way. I am contributing not just to the healthcare system but also to the entire Zionist enterprise, and I feel a euphoric sense that I have become a part of an historical movement.

ALTHOUGH MY JOB IS IN JERUSALEM, when I moved to Israel I decided to live in Tel Aviv and endure the hour-long daily commute. Tel Aviv is commonly, and not always kindly, referred to as "the bubble" because it can feel so insulated from the chaos and conflict that seem to dominate the rest of the country. A vibrant, dynamic mix of Mediterranean and Western, it is the Middle Eastern version of the city that never sleeps. I was also drawn to Tel Aviv's large expat community. In Tel Aviv, I feel engaged with the modern, forward-looking side of the country, the Israel that is known and admired throughout the world for its dozens of high-tech industries, the Israel glowingly portrayed in Dan Senor and Saul Singer's book, *Start-up Nation.*

But in Jerusalem, interacting with Lena and her family, I also feel engaged, albeit in a different way. Jerusalem, with its Jewish, Christian, and Muslim holy places, seems to me more like the Israel I had grown up learning about in my Conservative Hebrew day school in Connecticut. I also have many fond memories of the summers I had spent in Jerusalem as a child, with my parents and my younger brother and sister. But now, more than twenty years later, as a new immigrant, I get the sense that Jerusalem is becoming more and more defined by its Orthodox Jewish population. In Tel Aviv I keep running into old friends, including some who are Modern Orthodox, who have relocated from Jerusalem, complaining that it lacks the energy of Tel Aviv and that the religious atmosphere and poverty there are becoming unbearable. I sense that Jerusalem would be better suited to a more observant and settled-down version of myself; for now the buzz of Tel Aviv feels right for me. When I attended medical school in Tel Aviv in the mid-1990s, I discovered Tel Aviv's exciting social and cultural scene; it was as though a version of New York had been transplanted onto Israel's Mediterranean coast. Now as a single guy in my mid-thirties, I definitely prefer spending my nonworking hours here. On the other hand, Jerusalem echoes with thousands of years of history; every rock and tree is rich with meaning. It is in Jerusalem that I feel I am earning my place in the larger, historical Zionist mission. By dividing my time between Jerusalem and Tel Aviv, I feel like I am straddling the two great realities of Israel: the city that encompasses the ancient, rich roots of our people, and the city that embodies the glories of the modern State of Israel.

The daily drive to work, though in some respects a hassle, captures this for me, and sometimes in my car I am overwhelmed with what I acknowledge is a corny but deeply moving sense of my place in the sweep of history. Leaving the ancient port of Jaffa behind me, from which Jonah fled from God's summons only to be swallowed by a whale, I drive toward Jerusalem, passing through the Ayalon Valley, where the Bible tells us that Joshua asked the sun and moon to stand still, then past the old British police fortress at Latrun, which was converted after its capture during the Six-Day War in 1967 to the Armoured Corps Memorial and Museum, and then through the narrow pass of Sha'ar Ha-Gay (Bab el-Wad in Arabic), a critical point in the Arab siege of Jerusalem during the War of Independence in 1948. On the return trip, after a hard day at the hospital, the coastal plain unfolds in front of me, with the lights of Tel Aviv sparkling in the distance under the setting sun.

I FIND MYSELF THINKING ABOUT LENA as the days pass between our initial meeting and her follow-up appointment, and I wonder what is going on in her head. Has she told her sisters, her teachers, her friends? I'm busy settling into my new job and meeting new patients, but all the while I'm anticipating Lena's return. I look forward to starting her therapy and, I hope, getting her on the road to a cure.

But Lena and her parents don't show up for their appointment. No phone calls, no messages, nothing. After many attempts, the social worker finally reaches Lena's mother by phone and gets a vague excuse as to why they missed the appointment. Over the next two weeks we get a series of excuses for their ongoing absence: a family wedding, a test at school, a sibling sick at home. Finally, it comes out. They have become convinced that Lena's leg will be have to be amputated, and they are paralyzed by the mere thought of it. Mickey has already shared with me his suspicion that this was the reason for their nonappearance, and while I sputter in disbelief and bemoan the delay in starting treatment, he seems unruffled and takes it in stride. He tells me about a former patient, a Palestinian child whose father declared that he'd rather have a dead daughter than a daughter without a leg. The thought nauseates me. What could possibly drive someone to say that about his own child? Is their cultural fear of disfigurement so strong? How can concern about social devaluation and the possibility of not marrying off a child be so strong as to make her death preferable? Just as I am feeling the excitement of belonging, of fitting into my new home, I am acutely aware of how foreign this place is. In America, the parents' response was usually extreme, too, but in the completely opposite direction. Most families in the United States did not even want to wait for the chemotherapy to run its months-long course. They just wanted their child's tumor out, as quickly as possible. Why play games, they would ask? A child can live without a limb. And I could understand the impulse behind this. There is a life-threatening tumor in your child's body, and you want it removed immediately, whatever the cost. It seems intuitive that the longer it remains there, the more dangerous it becomes. It took time to explain to families that starting treatment with chemotherapy is an important step in eradicating any tumor cells that may already be circulating in the body, away from the site of the tumor and undetectable on MRIs (magnetic resonance imagings) or PET (positron-emission tomography) scans. That limb-sparing surgery would not increase the overall risk of a recurrence. But this is new for me, the experience of having a family refuse to bring their child in to begin treatment for fear of an amputation that is still very theoretical and unlikely to be necessary.

We offer to meet with Lena and her family to go over everything again, to explain the importance of getting started, and to reemphasize the likelihood of cure. But all of our cajoling via the social worker doesn't seem to help. There must be some magic word I'm not saying, some key that could unlock the box in which all their fears and frustrations are stuck. Still basking in the glow of my new citizenship, I may feel that at last I belong to this incredible place, but there is clearly still so much for me to figure out.

2

Off the Map

I T'S JULY 2006, and I'm in the departure lounge in the Guatemala City airport, returning to the United States from a vacation. A static-filled television proclaims that war has broken out between Israel and Hamas fighters based in Gaza. I had finished my training as a pediatric oncologist exactly one year earlier, had joined a well-established medical practice, moved into a spacious apartment in the suburbs with my girlfriend, and paid off my medical school debts. I seemed to be well on the road to a comfortably settled adulthood. But then, over the course of that year, I broke up with my girlfriend, moved into a smaller, more modest apartment, and discovered that private-practice medicine probably wasn't a good fit for me. I was also facing a growing crisis of faith. I had grown up in suburban Connecticut in a fairly observant Jewish home, the oldest son of a Conservative rabbi. I attended a Jewish day school, where Judaism and Israel-oriented topics composed a significant part of the curriculum, through the seventh grade. In college I majored in religious studies despite my father's wry, self-deprecating warning that I would discover that everything about religion is either made up or stolen. But despite learning during the course of those studies that his joke might not be that far off from the truth, I'd always maintained a fair degree of religious observance. Even after questioning the roots of my religious traditions, perhaps even because of that questioning, I felt that I emerged from my studies all the more engaged with and nurtured by my faith. Though I ate at nonkosher restaurants, I limited myself to vegetarian food. Though I turned lights on and off and watched television on the Sabbath, I didn't use the phone, travel by car, or write, and for the most part I stayed home for a quiet observance of the day of rest. I attended synagogue on many, if not most, Sabbaths, and always on holidays.

Working in pediatric oncology challenged all that, as I increasingly felt that my daily experiences were at odds with what I had always held true about the place of religion in the world. The constant exposure to suffering and death meant it no longer felt safe or comforting to hear that "things happen for a reason" or that "things work out in the end." What I saw every day at work belied such silly platitudes. About 75 to 80 percent of children with cancer do survive (counting all forms of cancer together), but that still means that almost one out of four children diagnosed with cancer dies.

During my general pediatric residency, my exposure to patient deaths was modest. This is not to say those children's deaths didn't affect me, but I could somehow rationalize them away by mentally isolating them as rare exceptions. After three years in general pediatrics training, drawn to the challenges of caring for children with complex and life-threatening illness, I went on to a three-year fellowship in pediatric hematology-oncology. Despite the difficulty of working with such seriously ill and so many dying children, something about the work resonated with me. Part of it was the drama, the extreme situations and high stakes. The practice of medicine definitely involves a certain amount of ego, and I loved doing something that I knew was intimidating for many other doctors. But it was more than just that. There was a personal challenge inherent in the work as well. In the same way that I had studied theology in college in part because of the way it challenged my personal beliefs, the experience of working with extremely ill children and their families also inserted itself into my soul in a way that left me uncomfortable and thinking about how I lived my own life. It was during my fellowship that death, suffering, and the challenges of how to cope with them became a part of my daily routine. I had begun my general pediatric residency training in 1998, not long after the *New England Journal of Medicine* published what was then considered to be a breakthrough paper by Dr. Joanne Wolfe, a pediatric oncologist in Boston who would go on to become an important figure in the then emerging field of pediatric palliative care. Dr. Wolfe and her colleagues found that almost all children with cancer who died did so with significant and poorly managed suffering. My experience matched Dr. Wolfe's findings: the children who died did so uncomfortably, and even the children who survived experienced terrible suffering in the process of getting there.

This book is in part about those children who don't survive. But it's also about those who do survive, but in a manner that leaves them changed in ways that are hard for most of us to grasp. It's about children for whom things don't work out according to hopes or expectations. It's about their families, who are also changed forever, and the clinicians who care for them. And because it's set in Israel, one of the most complex places on earth, it's also about individuals, communities, and even entire nations for whom things don't work out according to hopes or expectations. And, ultimately, it's about how all of these experiences changed me and my own expectations.

.   .   .

DURING MY FELLOWSHIP, the pace of my training was frantic enough that I was largely spared (or prevented) from having to truly process any of the suffering I saw. The necessity of moving on and caring for the next child did not allow for much time to sit and reflect, so that my experience of patient death was broad but not so deep.

There were isolated moments here and there, sometimes shared with other clinicians, or even at times with the children themselves and their families, when time would slow down and there would be some mutual acknowledgment of the sadness, and sometimes even the beauty, of our shared experience. But for the most part, those moments were rare gems meant to be pocketed and privately treasured, and not openly displayed in front of others in the midst of training.

When the fellowship ended, I joined a much smaller pediatric hematology-oncology practice. I lasted a year there. The pace of the clinical work was slower, and there was now time to reflect. Though the number of dying children seen by the practice was much smaller than what I had experienced during my fellowship, each death seemed to land on me with a heavier thud. At one point my pent-up feelings about all of the suffering I had witnessed suddenly exploded, like one of those gag cans with a spring-loaded snake that leaps out when you loosen the lid. The deaths I witnessed that year, as well as the lived experiences of those who survived, were intense. There was the little girl with relapsed leukemia after a bone marrow transplant, whose strong-willed mother, despite our attempts to dissuade her, demanded more and more chemotherapy in the hope that something would work, until death ended the debate in the form of an overwhelming infection that filled her veins with an evil mix of chemotherapy, leukemia, and bacteria. A lovely four-year-old boy, with great maturity and an astonishing air of ownership over his fate, would proudly report in detail each week on how he was feeling until he ultimately succumbed to a vicious leukemia that refused to respond to any therapy. There was a six-year-old I never really got to know, because by the time I met him a brain tumor had destroyed most of his ability to interact. Somehow, through the steroid-induced puffiness and slurred speech, hints of the little boy still inside him came through. His parents showed up weekly with piles of scribbled notes and printed brochures about alternative treatments they had found on the Internet, desperately hoping that this time, finally, they would present us with something that held out a real chance for their son, something that we wouldn't be able to dismiss as worthless.

After I'd been in the practice for a year, I could feel myself struggling. I wasn't sure how my colleagues managed it. Did they compartmentalize, harden themselves to the suffering? Ignore the pain and somehow leave it behind at work? Or were they so secure in their faith that they found solace in God, or Jesus, or Buddha, or whoever they believed was looking out for these poor souls? Did anyone really believe, as I often heard someone whisper after a child's death, that "they are in a better place"? Whenever I would hear this, I would inwardly grumble that if I truly believed that, I would immediately go there myself.

The one time I ventured to ask a colleague if she believed in this notion of a better place, she quickly responded, "Of course!" and looked at me, surprised. A devout Catholic, she apparently firmly believed that Jesus was waiting to embrace the departed souls of these suffering children. And this was a person I thought I knew well, someone who I thought shared my experience of working in oncology. Embarrassed by my own cynicism, I waited a long time before I asked anyone that question again. I continued to struggle, though. Do things happen for a reason, to teach us lessons (in other words, is meaning derived)? Or is it just that human beings are capable of looking back on a tragedy and interpreting it in a way that allows us to make some sense of it and grow from it (in other words, is meaning constructed)? The issue of agency, of whether or not there is a conscious, causative force behind these terrible things we witness, or if we are simply subject to the blind laws of nature, felt critical to me in the face of so much suffering. Studying religion in college had been stimulating, but the real-world experience of being a pediatric oncologist was proving too much for me to bear. As one patient's father, a curmudgeonly old science professor, told me on learning of my background in religious studies, "Ah, well, I suppose you're now just doing applied theology." But the applied version was turning out to be a lot harder to get my head around than the classroom kind.

I turned to my father, in his capacity both as a parent and as a spiritual leader. How was I to make sense of all of the death and suffering? How was I to engage in this kind of work day after day, fully immersing myself in the lives of my patients and their families, and still maintain the structure of ritual and belief that I had constructed? The suffering and death of these children argued against religion's kind, powerful, and loving view of the universe and the omnipotent being that ran it. I needed to find an explanation for this, to make sense of it all, or I would have to find a career with less exposure to it.

My father's brutally honest answer, that he had no idea, was an acknowledgment that I had arrived at one of life's great existential questions and one of humanity's greatest challenges: to make sense of a world that all too often seems cruel and unjust. Theodicy, the attempt to explain how a good and all-powerful God can possibly allow evil to exist, tries to give us reasons why bad things happen to good people.

Recognizing the ancient roots of this question (there is even a clay tablet dating from 1600 BCE inscribed with what scholars call the Babylonian Theodicy), I resolved to take a closer look at how others have approached the problem. I loaded a backpack full of philosophy books and set out for two weeks in Guatemala, seeking a quiet place to get away and do some reading. Between excursions to explore the countryside, I claimed a favorite spot at a small café tucked into the crumbling Spanish colonial architecture of Antigua. There I would sit dripping sweat and drinking warm beers in the humid Guatemalan summer while poring over thick volumes, taking notes as I read.

Unsurprisingly, there was no epiphany, no moment of glorious insight. But what I did begin to find during those weeks was a sense of direction, or at least of mission. Realizing how many others had agonized over the same issues made me feel less alone. I had no sense of where my career was heading, no sense of what I wanted from my personal life, no sense of how my faith system would hold up, but I felt that at least I was on my way toward finding, if not *the* answer to the question of theodicy, then perhaps an answer that would work for me.

It was at the end of the trip, having not checked email or listened to the news for days, that I heard about the war in Israel. Sitting in the airport, I saw on television that an Israeli soldier had been kidnapped on the Gaza border. Shortly thereafter there had been an attack by Hezbollah on the Israeli border with Lebanon, and the Israel Defense Forces (IDF) were mobilizing on both fronts. This was all very worrying, and not for the first time did I think that my place was there, doing whatever I could to help. I had grown up in a Zionist home. I studied in classrooms where an Israeli flag hung side by side with the Stars and Stripes. Maps of Israel adorned the walls, and at least once a year we raised funds to plant trees in Israel. I had spent a great deal of time there, starting with summers as a child, then visiting more and more often and for longer periods from high school into my college years. To top it all off, I had lived in Tel Aviv through all four years of medical school. My sister had already made aliyah, as had my brother, who, feeling a similar sense of duty, deferred law school in the United States for two years in order to volunteer to serve in the IDF. So it was not crazy that the oldest Waldman sibling was now considering a similar move, and I knew I would have my parents' support. Whenever I had thought about making aliyah in the past, it had always been more of an abstract consideration. But now, already primed for a life change, I felt that the timing was right. The struggle of the Jewish state resonated deeply with my own internal struggle. When I arrived back in the United States, I decided that the next step on my journey would be a move to Israel. I'm sure this came as a surprise to many of my colleagues. Most of the physicians I trained with followed fairly traditional paths of slow but steady advancement in academia. But I already sensed that this path was not going to work for me, that in my search for a sense of identity and place I needed to depart from the usual track. Where better to explore my faith and identity than in the country that I had been raised to think of as my other home?

PRIOR TO MY OFFICIAL ALIYAH in March 2007, I'd had a number of preparatory meetings with Jewish Agency officials in New York. Their job was to help organize my paperwork and make sure I would be greeted at the airport, as all new immigrants are, with a warm Zionist "welcome home." This was meant literally: I was told that someone from the Jewish Agency's offices in Israel would be there at the airport, on the arrival ramp before the customs area, holding up a sign with my name on it. This person would set up my new immigrant's benefits package and give me my national identification card. At my last meeting with the Jewish Agency representatives in New York, they gave me my one-way plane ticket and a letter to present on arrival, and they wished me well. On the appointed day, I excitedly headed to my new home. My parents saw me off at the airport, already talking about when they might make the move to Israel as well.

I arrived on a rainy spring morning to a homecoming that was not quite what I had anticipated. As I walked down the arrival ramp at Lod Airport, tired from the eleven-hour flight but beaming with pride, I scanned the area looking for the promised welcome-home sign. Not seeing anyone, I queried one of the customs agents, who testily directed me upstairs to the immigration offices, where the staff was just getting settled in for the day. The clerk helping me apologized as she shuffled through piles of paperwork without finding anything with my name on it. She finally gave up and just started filling out all the forms from scratch. A short time later I was on my way in a taxi to Tel Aviv, Israel's newest immigrant. My welcome hadn't been the triumphant return to Zion I had imagined, but no matter, I had arrived. And the bureaucratic hiccup on entry was even a bit charming, in a "you've gotta love this place" sort of way.

But as I began to settle in, I realized that my frustration with the government agencies that were supposed to be helping me had only just begun. Not long after my arrival I received a short letter outlining subsidies I might be eligible for, including a modest monthly stipend to get me started, and a notice about tax discounts I could apply for on major purchases, such as a car. But other than that, in contrast to the warm sales pitches about the glories of aliyah that I had been receiving from the Jewish Agency representatives back in New York, I felt that the powers that be had turned suddenly cold and uncaring. I heard nothing further until a letter arrived about a year into my new life as an Israeli, curtly informing me that I was being drafted into the army. This all certainly came as a bit of a surprise. I don't know what I had expected, and I certainly didn't need any coddling. I knew that many others had made aliyah under far more difficult circumstances. But for me as an individual, this move to Israel was momentous. It took a while for me to get used to the idea that the government's lack of interest in the ease of my acclimatization, or *klitah,* was not personal, but that in the eyes of the system I was just another individual who had decided to move to Israel. I wasn't a refugee fleeing religious persecution or the struggling remnant of a dwindling Jewish community in a hostile country. I was just another upper-middle-class American

Jew who had decided to relocate. I felt that I had made some significant career sacrifices to be here and that I deserved at least a
"thank you." Instead, I got "Get in line."

Even within Hadassah, where the hospital's bureaucracy was
just as bad as the government's, the opacity of the system left me
experiencing a constant low level of uncertainty, a vague sense
that I was missing out on something. My dealings were almost
entirely with Mickey, and while I was completely confident in his
honesty and interest in my well-being, I was never completely
sure whom I was dealing with higher up the ladder, and where
I stood with them. Things that in the United States were clearly
laid out in contracts, such as being reimbursed for attending professional conferences, became byzantine trials of emotional and
psychological endurance at Hadassah, where the rules seemed
to shift on a daily basis. My monthly pay stub was indecipher-
able beyond the fact that the numbers never seemed to match
from paycheck to paycheck. I wasn't even sure if I had actually
signed a formal employment contract with Hadassah; I certainly
hadn't been presented with or negotiated any terms of employment. I had simply been offered a position by Mickey and—in
part because I was still fresh out of training and didn't know any
better, and in part because I assumed this was simply how things
were done in Israel—I accepted the offer, which was accompanied by a handshake and the all-purpose *"yih'yeh b'seder"* ("it will
be okay"), which I took at face value. The saving grace was the
Pediatric Hematology-Oncology Department staff. The doctors,
nurses, and administrative staff embraced me as if I were a member of their own family and very quickly made the department
feel like home for me. Meanwhile, the larger medical system at
Hadassah remained indifferent to my existence, an indifference
that my bruised ego struggled not to take personally.

The crowning indignity occurred when the Ministry of
Health refused to grant me a license to practice medicine in
Israel, which was of course the reason I had made aliyah in the

first place. I had started work mostly as an observer, unable to function as a fully independent physician without first obtaining the Israeli license. I was allowed to "see" patients but couldn't do essential things like order chemotherapy or perform standard procedures like bone marrow aspirates or spinal taps. I had tried to obtain the license in advance of my arrival, but it was explained to me that it could not be applied for without a national identification number, and one receives a number only after one arrives in Israel and officially becomes a citizen. In short, there is no way to arrange for the license in advance. Once you are able to submit your license application, the process can take at best weeks and at worst months, during which time you of course cannot work as a physician. So you wait in limbo while the Health Ministry processes your papers, though Hadassah was at least letting me work in a limited capacity while I waited. The complication in my case, I was told at the time of the refusal, was that because I had attended medical school in Israel but then returned to the United States for my licensing exam, I was now required to take the same licensing exam that Israeli medical students take on graduating from medical school. It was as though my ten years of training, board certification, and professional practice as a senior physician had never happened. I filed an appeal with the Health Ministry, arguing that it would be absurd to examine me now on material I'd learned ten years earlier—basic science that I hadn't been using for years. If anything, I should be tested on the clinical skills and knowledge that I would need to have at my current level of practice. As the weeks dragged on while I waited to hear from the Health Ministry, I had moments of such frustration and disappointment that I considered giving up and going back to the United States. I kept telling myself that over the past decades many immigrants—including scientists, doctors, musicians, and academicians—had come to Israel under much more difficult circumstances and had to start all over again at the bottom of their professions in a new country and a new language. I hadn't exactly expected a red carpet to be rolled out for me, but the bureaucratic indifference, the apparent cruelty, left me unsettled.

Then, after weeks of waiting in increasing despair, an Israeli friend gave me my first lesson in how things get done in Israel. She mentioned my story to an afternoon radio talk show host who ran a popular segment that tried to help out ordinary people who were being taken advantage of by government bureaucrats, big corporations, etc. They interviewed me briefly on the air and tried also to have an on-air phone conversation with a representative from the Ministry of Health, who angrily hung up on them. That was on a Thursday afternoon, just as the Israeli weekend was starting. First thing Sunday morning (the first day of the workweek in Israel), I received a call from someone from the Education Ministry. The spot on the show had gotten some attention. The education minister wanted me to know that they were going to be in close contact with me until this matter was cleared up and that I shouldn't worry, as they now saw the absurdity of the situation. They would process my licensing papers as quickly as possible. Which was in fact what happened, to my considerable astonishment and relief.

Putting all of this behind me and finally able truly to get to work, I dive into my new job at Hadassah. I am still in awe of the physical surroundings. Looking out at the valley of Ein Kerem in southwestern Jerusalem, where Hadassah's main campus is located, with its eponymous stone-clad village nestled at one end, it's not hard for me to imagine how it must have looked two thousand years earlier, when John the Baptist was born there. I drive along the winding roads above the valley on my way to work in the early morning, and often, through the dissipating mist, I see a jackal, having finished a night of foraging, crossing the road. Sometimes I come upon an exhausted-looking group of soldiers navigating their way back to base after a night of field exercises. I'm never quite sure what century I'm in. The various

mosques and churches scattered throughout the valley, including the magnificent onion-shaped golden domes of the Russian
Orthodox church that sits on a slope just above the village, all
testify to the different religious traditions that have staked their
claim to this land over the millennia.

About two-thirds of the way down that slope sits the Hadassah Medical Center, a jumble of concrete buildings erupting from
the otherwise verdant landscape. What in the early 1960s must
have appeared as a great leap forward, a tribute to cutting-edge
science, medicine, and architecture in the proud new Jewish
state, now appears dusty and worn. On the highest peak above
the valley, perched above the hospital, stands a somber-looking,
unadorned square building, a military base that looks down
toward the west at the hospital and the village of Ein Kerem and
toward the east at what had been the pre-1967 border between
Israel and Jordan (the "Green Line"). Past that border, the Palestinian towns of Beit Jalah and Bethlehem can be seen at a distance. Surrounded by an imposing fence, the building is no more
than a dark glass-and-stone cube, silent and inscrutable, topped
by a cluster of antennae and satellite dishes. When I ask about
it, I'm never given a direct answer, just evasive responses—that
it's some sort of listening post for army intelligence. I can never
tell if the people being evasive are doing so because they are in
on some secret that I'm not yet Israeli enough to be a part of, or
if they are just acting like they are in on the secret because they,
too, don't really know. At hospital staff meetings, my habitual
seat at the conference table gives me a clear line of sight out the
window and up the hill to the base. I often look up during meetings and wonder what's going on up there, conjuring images of
daring exploits of military intelligence. I strain to pick out any
activity around the building, any hint of what might be happening inside it. In my fertile imagination it's filled with gleaming
banks of computers and massive video screens, with elite intelligence officers directing secret operations in our defense. I can't

help but wonder what the Palestinian families on the other side
of the hill think when they look up at it.

TO GET INTO THE HADASSAH MEDICAL CAMPUS you
pass through a gate where a guard briefly inspects you, and then
you try to find a parking spot among the terraced lots that cas-
cade down the hillside below the main complex. Leaving the
parking area on foot, you enter the lower level of a small shopping mall attached to the hospital and make your way up the
escalator, past the coffee shops with their trays of pastries laid
out for the morning rush, and out into the central plaza of the
medical complex. The Mother-Child Building, which houses all
of pediatrics in addition to labor and delivery, is to the right. The
ground floor is usually still pretty deserted when I get in; at this
early hour very few patients have arrived yet. The lobby is open
all the way to the top of the building, creating a soaring atrium
that rises up through the core. Each floor, open to this central
space, feels connected to the others, and by the middle of the
day you can watch staff and patients moving about on all the
floors at once, creating the sense of a buzzing beehive of activity.

The Pediatric Hematology-Oncology Department occupies
the beautiful, newly refurbished fifth floor, which was completed
just after my arrival. The department is shaped a bit like an excla-
mation point laid flat, with the central atrium sitting in the space
where the line hits the dot. The dot is where our offices are; the
line is the patient-care side, which is further divided into two
parallel hallways. The hallway on the right leads into the day
clinic. At the start of this hall are the physicians' exam rooms.
Farther down are two large bays, each of which is ringed with
patient beds separated by curtains, and with a central table for
children to play and do arts and crafts, or for parents to socialize.
The parallel hallway to the left houses the inpatient ward, with
eleven rooms that extend down the outer side. Both hallways

meet at the far end in a family lounge area with an enormous
floor-to-ceiling glass wall providing a view of the valley that can
only be described as biblical. The two hallways connect at three
other points: a staff room shared by the clinic and the inpatient
staffs, and two service spaces, both of which feel rough and
unfinished and often smell slightly of rotting food and gas. The
contrast between the polished, shiny main hallways and these
connecting spaces always makes me think of Paul Valéry's comment that God made everything out of nothing, but the nothing-
ness shows through. The unfinished aura emanating from those
spaces detracts from the beauty of the department, making it
appear somewhat incomplete, or as though decomposition has
already begun to set in.

WHAT MAKES THE PEDIATRIC hematology-oncology
department at Hadassah so special for me is the people. For all
of the social and cultural diversity that I had experienced in
New York, I am still overwhelmed by the diversity of both the
staff and patients at Hadassah. There are secular Israeli Jews; the
Modern Orthodox and the ultra-Orthodox Haredim, each with
their distinctive style of dress and traditions; Sephardic Jews
originally from North Africa and the Levant; immigrants from
Russia, Ethiopia, Europe, and the United States; Israeli Arabs and
Palestinian Arabs; religious settlers from the West Bank and left-
ists from the coastal plain; and medical tourists from the former
Soviet Union. Somehow, everyone manages to work together and
take care of one another. You are just as likely to find a Muslim
patient praying off in a corner on a small prayer rug as you are
to find a group of Jewish teenage volunteers and patients sitting
in a circle on the hallway floor having a few laughs. Arriving
early in the morning, I often find a parent sleeping on one of the
benches in the waiting area outside the offices, either someone
who had come in during the night with a sick child and was still

waiting for a room, or a Palestinian Arab who had woken up very early to make it in on time for an appointment, taking into consideration the amount of time it might possibly take to make it past military checkpoints. As the day progresses, the crowd milling throughout the department swells, a mélange of cultures, costumes, and characters you couldn't find anywhere else in the world. I love it all; this is my dream.

LENA'S FAMILY CONTINUES TO REFUSE to allow us to start her cancer treatment. The fact that this is spurred by an extremely theoretical fear of possible amputation at some point down the road is very hard for me to understand, especially as the alternative to treatment is death. I soon discover that this phenomenon is not limited to Muslims. Months later I meet Chaya, an eight-year-old girl from an ultra-Orthodox Jewish family who has been diagnosed with a rare connective tissue tumor in her foot. Because of the location and the tumor type, the treatment that offers the best hope for cure is to remove the foot in its entirety along with the tumor. Trying to be supportive, I point out to her parents that because this type of tumor is slow to spread and we appear to have caught it early, once the foot is removed Chaya will not need to receive any further treatment. This is a big deal, as the type of chemotherapy she would otherwise receive can be very poorly tolerated and the potential long-term side effects are not trivial. Chaya's parents, however, have other ideas. Over the next few weeks Chaya's father engages me in long hours of debate, entangling me in complex, Talmudic-style arguments in an attempt to get me to endorse any course of treatment other than amputation. As I try my best to navigate these discussions, I feel cornered. It's like being cross-examined on a witness stand. I am, after all, only human. I can only make what I believe to be the best medical recommendations in the strongest terms possible. I consult with colleagues, both in Israel and abroad, and the consensus is clearly in favor of amputation. But because this is such a rare tumor, I cannot say with 100 percent certainty that another course would be wrong. As one of my instructors used to say, medicine is not mathematics, and in medicine there is rarely such a thing as 100 percent certainty. And without it, I cannot, of course, compel Chaya's parents to take any course of action. Chaya's father finally manages to locate a surgeon abroad who is willing to try to remove the tumor while sparing the foot. The family hastily makes travel plans, informing our staff of their decision just as they are about to leave. I try not to feel personally dismissed. I send the father a note encouraging him to return to us for follow-up care after the procedure, and to feel free to contact us with any worries or concerns. I wish them luck, and very much hope that in the coming years their decision proves to be the correct one. But I can't shake the feeling of frustration that there is something in the calculus of these families, Arab and Jew alike, that eludes me. It's true that I am not myself a parent, but this is something bigger; there is some cultural element here that I just don't get.

Language is part of it. Though I spoke Hebrew fairly well before making aliyah, there is definitely room for improvement, especially in terms of the local slang and its use in the discussions I need to have with both staff and patients. The use of military jargon in the medical setting is particularly pervasive in Israel; almost everyone here serves in the military, and so military language becomes a sort of lingua franca in all aspects of life, a shared code that can be used for easy conversational shorthand. Having not yet been through my army service, I can't really understand much of the local slang.

In *Illness as Metaphor,* Susan Sontag writes of the dangers of using war and violence as metaphors when talking about illness. She warns against our tendency to objectify the patient and the illness, turning them into the "battlefield" and the "enemy" as we deploy our high-tech "weapons" against them. I try to avoid that kind of language, but sometimes these metaphors do indeed feel apt, perhaps less so when talking about patients but certainly when talking about the flow of the workday and the approach to workplace challenges.

"Captured territory is never relinquished," is one of the first phrases I learn, when we are discharging oncology patients from beds in the general pediatric ward, where they have been admitted because of hospital overcrowding. Those beds are listed as belonging to oncology patients, and if we are sending one of those patients home, we need to get another patient into that same bed immediately, before it can be reassigned to a non-oncology patient.

"Straighten the line," I hear several times a day, especially when things are hectic. This would be the equivalent of our saying in the United States, "Let's touch base" or "Let's make sure we're on the same page." The Israeli version references a combat situation; if the line of soldiers advancing in formation while firing on an enemy position becomes ragged and someone breaks formation and gets out ahead, he risks being accidentally shot by his own people. In our line of work, any breakdown in the prescribed order of things could also result in a loss of life. I'm not surprised to learn that the word for "pills," *cadurim,* is also the word for "bullets." There's just no escaping the military lingo.

Even as my Hebrew improves and I reach a comfortable level of fluency, I still have to contend with Arabic (not to mention the Russian that many of our patients from the former Soviet Union speak). When I started at Hadassah, I had some rudimentary Arabic and was able to say things like "Good morning" and "How are you?," even though I couldn't really understand the responses I would get. When I asked my first few Arab patients "How are you?," the reply was usually a simple *"Co'es."* I later learned that this means "okay" in Arabic, but because it also sounds similar to the Hebrew word for "angry," I spent the first few weeks shocked at how much rage appeared to be simmering beneath the surface in the hospital. Only after I mustered the courage to ask a colleague about this did I realize my mistake, and at the same time I learned a good lesson in the importance of precision in language in our complex environment.

OVER THE NEXT SEVERAL MONTHS I accumulate a roster of patients, each with his or her own challenges and charms. In addition to caring for patients who have been diagnosed with sarcomas, I also find myself frequently involved in the care of children, regardless of diagnosis, with other forms of advanced cancer, children who have relapsed multiple times or whose cancer has progressed despite treatment. Many of these children are still very functional, going to school, playing with friends, and enjoying life as much as possible. But by all measures they are children who will almost certainly die of their underlying disease, the question simply being when. Most of these children are being treated off-protocol, which is to say that no treatment map exists for them any longer. The protocols that we give families at the start of treatment really allow for only two possibilities: either the patient successfully completes the protocol, albeit at times with modifications, and becomes cancer free, or the patient has to stop the protocol because of intolerable side effects or because the disease is progressing despite therapy. So then what? In those latter instances we often try to mock up unofficial versions of third- and fourth-line therapies, which generally means using treatments that are not part of the standard protocol for that particular type of cancer. But realistically, in these situations nobody knows what, if any, treatment should be continued and, if so, at what dose and frequency. And with each relapse or failed treatment, clarity about how to proceed seems more and more elusive. Like many of my colleagues, I struggle with how best to manage these sorts of cases, and I am uncomfortable with the lack of a clear plan. And yet I love working with these patients.

Often, our guiding principle in managing children who are off-protocol, especially if their disease has progressed despite multiple therapies, is to try to provide them with as good a quality of life for as long as possible. But it is not always clear to me how children and their families decide what defines quality of life and how they still manage to have any faith in their floundering clinicians as they pursue that goal. For us, the crux of the issue remains the lack of protocol and the lack of formal guidelines. We struggle to create some sort of order in the chaos, to seek some wisdom that can inform our next move. We worry about continuing treatments that may be causing more harm than good, but at the same time the thought of stopping treatment is excruciating, an acknowledgment of failure. This is frequently compounded by the pressure from desperate parents to come up with something else, with anything that will halt the progression of their child's disease. "Doctor," they say, "try anything. What do we have to lose?" But there is always something more to lose, whether that means the child's continued suffering from the therapy's side effects, or ancillary damage to a body already wracked with disease, or, if the treatment actually hastens death, more time lost in a child's life. What is my responsibility to the child and what is my responsibility to the parents, and what do I do when the two seem to conflict? I am tormented by these situations, but somehow I find myself drawn to them again and again, searching for some way to navigate the uncertainty.

It occurs to me that in moving to Israel, in seeking to reinvent myself, I am also seeking my own protocol, my own sense of how to safely organize the universe around myself and to approach life's challenges. Maybe it's this uncertainty in my own life that draws me to these patients. In general, I'm all for adventure and for leaping into the unknown. But during the hard times, the scary times, the times when we feel lost and threatened, isn't a protocol what we all seek? A schedule, a set of rituals, a list of rules to follow that, as Rabbi Heschel might put it, will help us locate ourselves and guide us through to safety. The trick, of course, is that protocols cannot account for every exigency, cannot anticipate every response, not in oncology and not in life. For some people, the protocol that brings comfort may be a religious system, or simply a set of spiritual beliefs, or a diet and exercise regimen. For myself, I suppose I am hoping that in moving to Israel I will identify my own protocol—that my move to Israel *is* my protocol. I am convinced that I will find meaning and direction by integrating into Israeli society, by identifying which piece of the Zionist puzzle I represent. I'm sure that if I just take the necessary steps; learn the languages; pay my taxes; deal with the bureaucracy, the politics, the shared joys and sorrows, I will come out on the other end safe and sound.

TWO WEEKS AFTER OUR INITIAL MEETING, Lena's parents apparently have a change of heart. Lena returns to the clinic and gets started on treatment. She completes the osteosarcoma protocol with clockwork precision: chemotherapy, surgery (tumor removed, leg intact), more chemotherapy. She finishes about nine months after starting, and all of our expectations, all the statistics, point to the likelihood that she is cured. This is the sort of outcome that is deeply satisfying to all oncologists, the reason many of us go into this field. And so I am devastated when she returns two years later with a massive recurrence in her pelvic bones. The location of the recurrence precludes surgical removal, and there is not much in the way of treatments that can be offered with any realistic hope for cure. Despite the dismal prognosis we start a new chemotherapy agent, maybe as much for ourselves as for Lena and her family. After a brief window of improvement, the tumor quickly begins to grow again and then to spread, and we find ourselves with no protocol, no map, just the despair that comes with watching as this journey approaches its inevitable end.

. . .

AVI IS A TWELVE-YEAR-OLD BOY with Ewing's sarcoma, a
tumor that also tends to occur in bone. He was first diagnosed and
treated several years before my arrival at Hadassah and has had
several recurrences since then; by the time I become involved
in his care, he is receiving carefully calibrated off-protocol chemotherapy roughly every three weeks. I use the term "carefully
calibrated" when speaking with him and his family in the hope
that this lends the treatment some authority, some air of scientific validation. But the truth is that "calibration" simply means
we adjust the dosing and timing of each treatment based on how
well he tolerated the previous one. When his blood counts drop
too low one week and he is admitted with a dangerous infection,
we slightly decrease the next dose to try to avoid a similar epi-
sode. When he suffers severe nausea and mouth sores so painful that he can't even drink water for two weeks (a common,
unpleasant side effect of chemotherapy), we space out the timing
of his treatments by a few more days to allow for better recovery
between treatments. The goal is to keep the cancer at bay while
not causing too many side effects. In other words, to help Avi
maintain the best quality of life possible, for as long as possible.

I first meet Avi on a day when he is just dropping in for a
check of his blood count, something done routinely once a week
between treatments. The blood count helps us monitor the treatment's effect on Avi's immune system as well as make sure he
does not require transfusions of blood or platelets, both of which
can become dangerously low from chemotherapy. Red blood
cells are necessary for oxygen transport throughout the body;
platelets are part of the clotting system and help stop bleeding.
Transfusions of one or the other are not uncommon during the
course of cancer treatment and are usually not considered anything to get excited about. Mickey, who usually oversees Avi's
care, is busy today, and because it should be a quick visit he asks

me to step in for him. I pull aside the curtain from the corner of the bay that Avi has claimed this morning and find a thin, pale boy dwarfed by the overstuffed reclining chair that envelops him. Even though he's sitting, I can see how frail he is, his wispy body barely registering in the ill-fitting black trousers and white button-down shirt that look like they belong to an older brother and were grabbed from his closet by mistake that morning. He glances up only briefly, intently studying a religious tome open on his lap. On top of his pale head, bald from chemotherapy, sits a wide black velvet yarmulke. Dangling below it, on both sides of his head, appear to be *payos,* the sidelocks cultivated by extremely Orthodox Jews. They are tucked behind his ears, but the yarmulke sits just askew enough that I can see that the *payos* are fake and have probably been sewn onto his yarmulke by his mother, so that he'll look like all the other boys in his class. I am by now familiar with the variety of responses children may have to chemotherapy-related hair loss. During our initial conversations about treatment, they are often more focused on their hair loss than on anything else, despite our reassurances that their hair will grow back when the treatments are over. This is especially true of adolescents, who are frequently also grappling with normal teenage issues of appearance and self-image. Being bald myself, my standard line used to be that when their treatment is over their hair will grow back just the same, while I will still be stuck like this forever. But I dropped this line from my repertoire after one child tartly responded that she would rather be bald forever than have cancer.

Many children go through chemotherapy with no attempt whatsoever at hiding their baldness, hardly seeming to notice their lack of hair. Others choose to wear hats, or bandannas, or go so far as to wear a wig. This, however, is my first encounter with fake *payos* attached to a yarmulke. I assume they are an integral part of Avi's emerging religious identity, as important as studying his religious texts and preparing for his bar mitzvah.

I introduce myself, and though he nods hello with a slight smile, Avi eyes me warily. I am still self-conscious about my Hebrew, my thick American accent making clear that I am not a native. Avi's mother greets me warmly, with the deep half-bow that I by now recognize is a proxy for a handshake among deeply religious Jewish and Muslim women, for whom physical contact with men outside their family is forbidden. Despite her smile, I sense that she, too, is suspicious of me and disappointed that Mickey is unavailable. Avi, a veteran of these between-treatment visits, cuts to the chase: "Do I need a platelet transfusion?" I glance down at the printout of Avi's counts from blood drawn that morning, and it's a tough call. His platelet count is theoretically high enough that he doesn't need a transfusion, but as compared with previous weeks it seems to be falling at a rate that suggests it might be wise to go ahead and give him one just to be safe. As I start to explain my thinking, Avi makes a sour face and kicks back in his chair. He crosses his thin, pale arms and starts making that "tsk, tsk" clicking noise with his tongue that kids make when they are upset and trying not to cry. "But I have a trip with my class this afternoon. I'll never make it if I have to stay for platelets!" I hesitate. To change course now will risk appearing indecisive in front of Avi's mother. On the other hand, I don't want to be unduly rigid and end up alienating Avi. Besides, I admire his desire to preserve some degree of normalcy, to defend his right to some small pleasures.

I suggest a compromise. We can skip the transfusion today if he is willing to return for a check again tomorrow, and if he promises to return immediately today if he shows any signs of bruising or bleeding. The words are barely out of my mouth and he is already leaping up, grinning, yarmulke and fake *payos* flying off his head. The intravenous tubing that runs from his chest wall to the bag of fluids on the IV pole next to him is jerked tight in his excitement, almost pulling the pole down onto him. "Yes!" he shouts. Exuberant and wide-eyed below his hairless eyebrows, he sees his opening. "Can I go now?" Avi's mother looks at me, smiling. I let out a big internal sigh of relief.

I end up staying involved in Avi's care through subsequent visits. In crafting Avi's ongoing therapy, we base our plans as much as possible on case reports and on consultation with colleagues at hospitals both in Israel and abroad. I often turn to my old mentors from my fellowship in my search for guidance. But the reality is that when Avi's parents ask me how many courses of chemotherapy he will get, I simply can't answer. They want a protocol, a map. They want to know that after some specific number of courses, whether fifteen or five hundred, he will be okay, cured, able to return to being a normal kid. But at this point in Avi's treatment, any concept of a real protocol has long since vanished. He will continue getting chemotherapy either until his frail body can no longer tolerate it or, more likely, until the tumor reappears elsewhere in his body, demonstrating that it is no longer responsive to the current treatments. With each new ache, each slight fever, no matter how unremarkable, Avi's parents rush him to the clinic: *Is this his disease?* they ask. *Do we need to do more tests or scans?* Usually these aches and pains are nothing. But sometimes they do indicate a problem. When they turn out to represent a progression of his disease, we alter course, try a new drug or add some localized radiation. But with each recurrence we are farther and farther off-protocol, and we have fewer and fewer options left. It makes me think of one of those maps from the early age of exploration, the ones with wild beasts and sea monsters indicating the limits of the known world, and I know that at this point we're out there among the monsters. Now and then Avi's parents approach me with questions about new treatments they've heard of. The Internet is rife with people, many with less than noble intentions, offering false hope to families like Avi's. All Avi's parents want is to get him back on some sort of plan that might lead somewhere, to relocate him and themselves on a map. But in Avi's case there no longer is a map, and we blindly forge ahead through dark and uncertain seas.

One day in the clinic Avi approaches me waving an invitation to his bar mitzvah. As a rule I don't attend my patients' bar or bat mitzvahs because I worry that if for some reason I have to miss one, that patient and family will feel slighted. Jerusalem may be a city, but it feels more like a village. Everyone seems to know everyone, and everyone talks. But in Avi's case I make an exception. Something about the faith he has shown in me over the past few months, his willingness to allow me to negotiate his care with him, has left me feeling particularly grateful to him. I want to see him outside the hospital, celebrating his hard-won milestone. The bar mitzvah is beautiful, and Avi is radiant, grinning from ear to ear as he chants his Torah portion in front of the congregation, as if no other moment in time, nothing the future may bring, matters as much as this moment right now.

3

Borders

FEVERS DURING THE COURSE OF CANCER treat-
ment are not something to be taken lightly. Because of the
depressive effect that chemotherapy has on the immune system,
patients are extraordinarily susceptible to all sorts of infections.
Fever may herald the onset of some mundane, run-of-the-mill
cold, but it may also signal the start of a far more dangerous
infection, which could rapidly progress to become life threatening. In rare instances, patients can go from looking and feeling fine to being on life support or worse in a matter of hours.
Because of this danger, parents of children undergoing cancer
treatment are taught that at the slightest sign of fever, regardless
of time of day, they must bring their child in immediately for
evaluation and antibiotics. This can be tiresome for our young
patients, not to mention for parents balancing work with caring
for both a sick child and her healthy siblings. Already dealing
with the stress of cancer treatment, these children must come
in at the slightest sign of a fever, even if they feel fine, and be

hooked up to intravenous antibiotics. Then they sit here, bored, for however many days it takes for their blood counts to recover enough so that they can be safely discharged. With luck, they will have a few days off before being admitted for their next round of chemotherapy.

And so I find myself one Sunday evening during my pediatric hematology-oncology fellowship in New York on duty in my hospital's urgent care center, evaluating a ten-year-old boy with a recurrent, metastatic tumor who has just been brought in by his mother because he is running a fever. Sam's parents are Irish immigrants and still speak with a thick, and at times impenetrable, brogue. Sam is a good student, quiet and polite, always with a book in hand. His pale freckled face and the few wisps of reddish hair that still cling to his otherwise bald scalp bear witness to his heritage.

I know Sam from previous admissions. It's quiet this evening in the urgent care center and I feel pretty much on top of things, so while his mother steps over to the front desk to register, I sit with Sam to keep him company and make small talk. His vital signs are stable, and he's already hooked up to intravenous antibiotics. Although he looks pale, there's nothing about him that suggests that this will be anything other than a routine admission for fever and low blood counts. Sam is usually easy to talk to, quick to share his thoughts about whatever book he's reading lately (he's brought *Treasure Island* with him this time), but this evening he's very quiet. He seems distracted and won't look me in the eye.

"What's wrong?" I ask. "Is something bothering you or hurting you?"

I'm suddenly worried that Sam may be more ill than he appears. It's not unusual for children to have difficulty articulating their feeling that something is amiss. Often they will simply say that "something feels wrong," or that they feel dizzy, or out of breath, or scared, and it turns out that what they are really feeling are the signs of an impending severe infection or organ failure.

I watch Sam's face carefully, trying to read what may be going on inside. He maintains a sullen silence, but after some prodding he finally looks at me and barks, "I'm just *tired* of the hospital!"

Nobody wants to be admitted to the hospital for any reason and, unsurprisingly, many kids on chemotherapy eventually hit the point where reality and fatigue kick in. I've been through this sort of outburst before, so I launch into my usual routine. I remind Sam that I also wish he weren't being admitted, but that this admission is for his own safety, and that we can hope this will be just a short stay and that his blood counts will recover quickly. But the usual approach doesn't work. Sam, most likely even more annoyed by my patronizing adult tone of voice, looks at me, exasperated.

"It's *not* just this admission! I *know* my counts will go back up. This isn't my first time, you know. But as soon as my counts go up, that means I'll have to come back in a couple of days for the next treatment, and it never ends. I'm *not* getting better! I'm *tired* of the treatments!"

And then, an angry declaration: "I'm going to *die* anyway!"

I know he's not speaking metaphorically. All of my colleagues have their own stories about the surprising maturity and insight of children with life-threatening illness. The look on a young child's face as you are trying to put the best possible spin on a bad situation, a little boy's offhand comment, a little girl's gesture of disbelief—we've all experienced these heartrending moments. But the naked matter-of-factness of Sam's declaration is terrifying. With an understanding and an acceptance that is way beyond anything that his parents or his clinical team are capable of, this little boy knows he is going to die.

I am keenly aware of my own discomfort and unsure of how to respond. At this point I'm still in training and terrified of saying or doing the wrong thing—not just for Sam's sake but also for my own. I worry about how the more senior clinicians might react if they disapprove of my reply to Sam. In mere seconds I'm transformed from an assured young doctor, feeling like I can handle anything, to a nervous trainee wishing that the attending physician on call or a well-seasoned nurse would walk in and take over. The floodgates open at this point, and Sam continues to pour out his feelings. I can't decide if I'm praying for or dreading his mother's return. What if she thinks it was something I'd said that sparked this outburst? Even worse, it's Sunday, and aside from another young doctor on call in the department upstairs, I'm pretty much on my own. The attending physician on call is at home, and though I can page him, we're told to reserve these phone calls for pressing issues, and I'm not sure he will think this qualifies.

Near tears, Sam tells me how much he hates the chemotherapy, that he feels it's no longer doing anything but making him feel sick and making him stay in the hospital. Sam declares that he understands if he stops the treatments he will die (which is true), but he thinks this is going to happen soon enough anyway (hard to know but possible), so he would prefer to just stop now.

I try to imagine what someone with more experience would say. I ask Sam if he's talked about this with Dr. Connolly, his primary doctor, or with his parents, figuring if the answer is yes, I can just follow their lead and support whatever they've said.

"No," he says, "I don't talk about being sick with my parents because it just makes them sad. And Dr. Connolly doesn't really talk to me. I don't think he likes me."

I'm at a loss as to how to respond to *that,* but Sam's mother rescues me. The instant he hears her opening the door to the treatment room Sam goes quiet, a slight flush in his pale cheeks the only sign that anything has been going on. She tells me the paperwork is taken care of and, noticing the color in Sam's cheeks, puts a hand on his forehead to check for fever. She asks how long I think it might be until he is moved to a bed upstairs. Seizing the opportunity to escape, I excuse myself to check on the bed situation. I don't say anything in parting to acknowledge Sam's outburst, nor do I bring it up during the admission process. The next day I cautiously mention Sam's concerns to Dr. Connolly. He barely responds, not even looking up from the charts on his desk as he dismisses both Sam's anxiety and me. I am too timid to be more forceful or to take the initiative and try to talk with Sam's mother myself.

Several weeks and a few doses of chemotherapy later, a CT (computerized tomography) scan confirms that Sam's tumor is progressing despite the treatments. The decision is made to stop chemotherapy, focusing on Sam's comfort and the quality of however much life he has left. During fellowship training, most of our time is spent either in the inpatient ward or conducting laboratory research; fellows have very little exposure to the outpatient clinic, which is actually, if all is going well, where patients spend a majority of their time and where most of the big conversations happen. Because of this, I never find out how the process unfolds, what conversations take place between Sam and his parents. I see Sam in passing only one or two more times during brief admissions before he dies at home. Despite that one painful moment of honesty, we never really talk again about what is happening to him. I can't decide if it was cowardice that kept me from continuing that conversation with Sam, or if it represents a flaw in our medical training. But either way, his courage stands as a stark rebuke to my inaction.

Yes, it's hard to talk about death with our patients—whether they are adults or children. But shouldn't that be part of a doctor's job? Previous generations of doctors apparently didn't think so. At one time, Western medicine considered hiding information from patients to be not only acceptable but also possibly even beneficial. The American Medical Academy's first code of ethics, published in 1847, stated: "The life of a sick person can be shortened not only by the acts, but also by the words or manner of a physician. It is, therefore, a sacred duty to avoid all things which have a tendency to discourage the patient and to depress his spirits." It is often the case that a patient's well-meaning and protective family members feel pretty much the same way. I recall as a medical student watching the adult children of an elderly man about to be operated on for an abdominal tumor implore the surgeon not to tell him what was in his belly. Better, they said, to let him think that everything was okay and allow him to enjoy what time he had left free of worry. It is only relatively recently that Western medicine has shifted away from this sort of paternalistic model of care. In the United States, only since the late 1960s have surveys started to show that an increasing number of physicians are inclined to disclose bad news directly to their adult patients.

In pediatrics, the ethics of disclosing bad news to our patients is even more complex. Even as things began to shift in the world of adult medicine in the 1960s, the default at that time was still not to disclose bad news to children. It's only during the past two decades that there has been more of a movement to include children, in an age-appropriate manner, in discussions of bad news and medical decision making. Developmental stage is a major factor. At what age can children really understand the concepts of serious illness and death? Most studies suggest that by age nine most children have a concrete understanding of death as an external and permanent state. By age eleven, children with advanced cancer understand that their lives are at risk, and they actually want to be a part of the discussion of their illness. But for many parents and even clinicians there is a degree of magical thinking involved that is akin to what I had observed as a medical student with those adult children of that elderly patient: if a child doesn't know how truly sick he is, perhaps he will feel better. At the very least, he won't feel worse, won't lose hope. There is also, of course, the natural instinct of a parent to protect one's child. And, yes, something feels unnatural about having this sort of conversation with a child; children shouldn't be developing life-threatening illnesses. But the fact is that it happens, and a conversation with the child needs to take place—not simply a recitation of unpleasant facts or a relaying of scary information, but a dialogue in which we engage the child at her level of understanding, allowing her to ask questions, to control how much or how little she wants to know. We tell ourselves that we don't involve children in these conversations for their own good, that they're too young to understand anyway. That it's our responsibility to shoulder the burden and make the difficult decisions for them, with their best interests in mind. But what if, as the data suggest, these assumptions are all wrong?

When I joined a private practice and became an attending physician in the United States, I began to confront these issues from higher up on the ladder of responsibility. I never forgot that experience with Sam, and in part because of it I worked hard to try, whenever possible and at developmentally appropriate levels, to include my young patients in the conversations that I was having with their parents. But with many parents it's an uphill battle, and the small amount of confidence I began to develop in the United States dissolved in the face of the new cultural challenges I faced when I moved to Israel.

I am surprised, for example, to discover that working with the Haredi community is one of my biggest challenges here in Israel. I come from an observant—though not Orthodox—family, and I had Modern Orthodox and Haredi patients during my years of training back in the United States. When my American friends comment on how fascinating it must be to work with a Palestinian Arab population whose culture and sensibilities are so completely different than my own, I half-jokingly reply that there are times when I feel that I understand the Palestinians better than I understand the ultra-Orthodox Jews. They're no more or less friendly than parents from other backgrounds that I meet, but there is something more insular about them, a distance they impose in the course of our dealings that I don't experience with other types of Jews, or with Muslim or Christian families, for that matter.

MOSHE IS AN ELEVEN-YEAR-OLD BOY from an ultra-Orthodox community in Jerusalem who comes to us with a large mass just above his left knee. He is a charmer, and he has an impish streak that surely puts him at the center in any classroom or in schoolyard antics at his Haredi *cheyder.* With a mischievous glint in his eye and a crooked grin, he manages at every visit, no matter how he is feeling, to make a joke—often at my expense—that cracks both of us up.

Moshe's parents know that we suspect he has cancer—the enormous mass is impossible to ignore—but I wait until after we have completed the initial workup tests and have received the biopsy results confirming the diagnosis of osteosarcoma before I have Moshe and his parents come in so that we can discuss the findings. I first sit alone with his parents, breaking the news to them and letting them know that I would like to include Moshe in the conversation we are about to have about his diagnosis and treatment. I reassure them that I will speak carefully and in a manner that is developmentally appropriate. At first they hesitate and ask that we just say he has an "illness," perhaps a virus, and that he will get better, but after some discussion we reach a compromise. They ask me not to use the term "cancer," which I agree to unless he himself brings it up. But they do give me permission to discuss the treatments and not simply wave this whole thing off like it's some sort of minor infection. Meanwhile, Moshe has been sitting out in the waiting area surrounded by children who are bald and obviously ill. Many of the kids are walking around with IV poles from which bags full of brightly colored medicine hang, with tubing that snakes down and runs under their sleeves and collars. Moshe is no dummy, and within minutes of walking into the room, I am sure that he already has it all figured out.

I engage Moshe delicately, referring only to a "sickness" in his body, mainly in his leg, that we need to treat. I explain that he will get medicine, some via IV and some by mouth, and that he will also need surgery on his leg. At no point do I say explicitly how dangerous the sickness is. And Moshe doesn't ask. He politely listens, nods, and says no when I ask if he has any questions. I feel like I'm being a bit dishonest, but this is one of our first meetings, and I'm still trying to get a sense of his developmental stage and maturity. And, of course, I have his parents hovering off to the side, watching intently, gauging how much they can really trust me. I tell myself that the conversation will develop over time.

Moshe's tumor responds well to the initial chemotherapy, visibly shrinking, and after three months he is transferred to the surgical department to have it removed. In many types of pediatric cancer, neither systemic chemotherapy nor surgical removal alone is sufficient for the patient to be cured. What is needed is a combination of local control (treatment focused on destroying or removing the primary tumor itself) and systemic chemotherapy (to eradicate any tumor cells that may have already spread but that may be too small to be detected and surgically removed). Local control usually means surgery, radiation, or a combination of the two. But osteosarcoma isn't particularly sensitive to radiation, so in Moshe's case complete surgical removal is critical. Unfortunately, Moshe's tumor has crossed into the knee, so this is one of the rare situations where the only way to ensure complete removal of the tumor is to amputate his leg. Moshe bears this news with a display of resolve, even forcing a smile; like many Orthodox Jews, he peppers his speech liberally with exclamations of "God willing" and "with God's help," even when faced with terrible news. I wonder bitterly to myself where God's help was when Moshe was diagnosed with bone cancer, but I suppose it's this faith that helps him maintain his positive outlook and his belief that he will successfully complete the treatment protocol and be completely cured.

After the surgery Moshe gets a break for several weeks to allow for the wound to heal before resuming the rest of his planned chemotherapy. Because of the delay, I order a repeat CT scan of his chest, a common site of metastasis, before resuming the chemotherapy. I'm dismayed to find multiple metastatic lesions, small tumors scattered like seeds throughout his lungs. In the few minutes it takes to read a CT scan, Moshe's prognosis has gone from fairly good to near-certain death. Because the tumor has spread despite standard chemotherapy, there is little hope that any other treatments will be more effective. And there is no way surgically to remove all of the tumors visible on the scans, let alone the many more that must be there that are too small for us to detect. A biopsy is arranged to confirm the CT findings, and this time I accede to his parents' request and explain to Moshe that the procedure is for something in his lungs that we are unsure of, maybe an infection. It's only a white lie, since strictly speaking it is true that this really could be anything. But, realistically, I know the odds are against us and that in doing more tests we are just delaying the necessary conversation. The biopsy confirms the progression of Moshe's cancer. Though I discuss the results with his parents, I agree not to explain the full import of this to Moshe, mentioning only that we will be changing the type of chemotherapy he is getting and hoping that he doesn't press us to explain why. Despite our hope that a change in agents will lead to at least an improvement, after several courses of the additional chemotherapy we find that the tumors are only growing larger. There are no more treatment options left.

I can no longer avoid the conversation or hide the truth in white lies. Looking at the CT scan, I remember Sam and think about how I will break this news to Moshe, what his reaction might be, and how I might respond. That there will have to be some sort of conversation is clear: Moshe has been avidly following along on a copy of his protocol, crossing off treatments week by week and counting the days until he's done. Completely stopping therapy in the middle of the protocol will not go unnoticed. And he's a bright kid. He's already acting like he knows something is wrong, already suspicious of the change in chemotherapy and the additional days it added to his treatment plan. I meet with his parents privately and lay it all out for them. I estimate that Moshe has about two to three months left, though oncologists are notoriously bad at that sort of prognostication. His father, a burly man with an enormous bushy beard and *payos,* stares at me impassively, inscrutable. I wait for him or his wife to say something, or to start crying, or to reach for each other—to react to this terrible news in some way. But they remain stony-faced and stoic. There is almost an air of dismissiveness toward me, and I feel the familiar insecurity that occasionally grips me in what is still for me a foreign environment. Do they not believe me? Are they waiting to hear from someone older and more experienced, or with better Hebrew? Or is this how their faith starts to kick in? Just as Moshe's faith allowed him to accept the amputation, maybe this is simply their way of internalizing, of adjusting to the news. I have been, I think, perfectly clear. There is no further chemotherapy we can offer with a realistic hope for a cure. Moshe will ultimately die of his disease, and we will do all we can to support him and to make that process comfortable. Moshe's parents continue to sit there, speechless. Maybe I'm just not being sensitive enough to the cultural differences between us, or perhaps they are simply in shock. When I see that no further meaningful discussion is going to happen that day, I schedule a meeting for the next day, thinking that they need time to collect their thoughts, consult with their rabbis, digest the new information. The one thing I ask in the meantime is for permission to speak with Moshe now, in their presence, to let him know that there will be some changes in the treatment plan and to gently begin to introduce the idea that things may not be unfolding as planned. The impassiveness instantly dissolves. "Absolutely not!" is the clear, angry response from both Moshe's father and mother. I try to assuage their concerns, explaining the data we have accumulated on children and end-of-life decision making. Their response is an unequivocal no.

I decide to defer the issue of what to say to Moshe until the next day's meeting, hoping that overnight they will change their minds. Maybe they will even broach the subject with him themselves, in a way that is more in tune with their own cultural mores. But at our meeting the next day they again refuse even to entertain the idea of allowing me to speak with Moshe about his recurrence. "Why does he need to know?" his father says, again with a hint of anger. "It will only add to his stress. Let him live his life, be happy, and whatever happens, happens. Only God knows what will happen. Not you, not us. We don't decide. Just God."

I can't argue with that. And as Mickey often reminds me, when religious parents are left with the option of being angry with God or angry with us, guess who they pick? I briefly consider speaking with Moshe anyway, at some point when I'm alone with him. Don't I have a responsibility to him? To not leave him like Sam, scared of what he knows inside but what no one is willing to say? But I fear that this would rupture my increasingly tenuous relationship with his parents, and that a further loss of trust might hinder my ability to provide care as his disease progresses. I also have to consider the fact that, in the end, no matter what we do Moshe will die and his parents will be left to continue their lives. I don't want to leave them with the sense that they failed to protect him—from the tumor or from me—in his time of need.

So we negotiate. I promise to respect their wishes, but I also tell them that I do not want to lie to Moshe—ever. I agree to their request that I not initiate the conversation with Moshe about his prognosis, and I promise that I will not try to elicit from him his thoughts or concerns. But if he starts the conversation of his own volition, if he asks me what is happening to him, I reserve the right to answer truthfully. Moshe's parents agree, but not without a final disdainful "You'll see. He won't ask." They throw me a dismissive look on their way out, as if *I'm* the one who doesn't understand what is going on here. Maybe they're right.

Weeks pass, during which I continue to see Moshe regularly at the clinic, both to monitor him for symptoms and to convey the message to him and to his parents that he is still a part of our system, that we are there to support him. We start him on a regimen of daily oral chemotherapy pills, which at best might slow the cancer but which in all likelihood just serve to maintain the pretense that Moshe is getting treatment. Oral hope, Mickey calls it. Of course, I hope each week that he will ask me what is happening to him. He must be wondering why he is not getting IV chemotherapy anymore and why his treatments seem not to be having any of the usual side effects. But he says nothing. He does stop asking to see his protocol, which I interpret as an awareness on his part that something has changed. A few times I edge close to the line I've carefully drawn with his parents, vaguely baiting him, hoping he will give me an excuse to start the conversation though never pushing hard enough to feel that I am violating my promise. But even when his slight cough turns into a deeper, more persistent rattle, and when that turns into shortness of breath requiring him constantly to have an oxygen tank by his side, Moshe never asks me anything. Toward the end of his life, when it no longer makes sense to burden him with coming to the clinic each week, Moshe's parents agree to have one of our nurses help care for him at home, where he dies quietly one afternoon. The nurse calls to let me know and asks me to come to the apartment to pronounce him dead.

I pull up across the street from the building and as I exit

my car I feel as though every single person in the neighborhood has stopped to stare at me. It's clear I don't belong here, with my chinos, rolled-up shirtsleeves, and bare head easily marking me as an outsider in this ultra-Orthodox enclave. Everyone here knows that Moshe has been ill, and from the stethoscope hanging out of my pocket it must be clear who I am and why I have come. I put my head down and hurry into the apartment building. This neighborhood is just a few minutes' drive from Hadassah, around a bend in the valley, and as I cross the street I catch a glimpse of the hospital in the distance. But despite the proximity, I feel like I've just gotten out of my car in another country, another world.

The door to the apartment is ajar, and the living room is already filling with men, one of whom waves me down a short hallway to a back bedroom. When I enter I barely recognize the gray, emaciated body of the boy lying there. I kneel by the bedside, putting a hand on his thin forearm. I silently apologize to him. There is a window open above the bed, and a hot wind blows in, carrying with it the sounds of children playing outside in the street. From somewhere across the valley there is the persistent ratcheting of a jackhammer, metal clanging on stone, man tearing into the ancient landscape, the sound of a city's growth while here all has gone still.

As I go through the formalities of declaring Moshe dead, I replay the course of his illness in my mind, reviewing how I had managed the issue of communication. Although it wasn't wrong to allow Moshe's parents to maintain some measure of control, some sense that they were acting in the best interests of their son psychologically and emotionally, perhaps I gave in too easily, scared off by the huge culture gap between us. And so did I leave Moshe feeling abandoned and thinking that I didn't care about him, as Sam had felt about his doctor? Or, unfamiliar as I was with this family's values, was I wrong in assuming that Moshe needed to have this conversation with me? Such a smart kid, and he never asked me a thing. It occurs to me that this may have been intentional. We advocate for a patient's right to know about his own medical condition, but what about the patient who may want to exercise the right *not* to know?

As I pass through the living room on my way out of the apartment, I see Moshe's father, who is praying with a cluster of men from the neighborhood. I pause to convey my condolences and to say goodbye. He barely looks up. Contrary to my usual practice, I don't visit Moshe's family during the week of shivah, telling myself it's because I have already said my goodbyes. But I know that I'm also avoiding confronting my own conflicted feelings. Mickey, braver than I, goes. He tells me that after sitting silently for a while, ignored by Moshe's father, he rose to leave, only to have Moshe's father suddenly look up and angrily say, "So, you people still believe we should have told him?"

MOSHE'S ULTRA-ORTHODOX NEIGHBORHOOD is not the only alternate universe just a stone's throw from the hospital; the same can easily be said of the towns and villages in the West Bank areas governed by the Palestinian Authority (PA). The Green Line, the border established between Israel and Jordan when the armistice agreements were signed in 1949, is just a few minutes' drive from the hospital. From the top of the hill, just alongside the army base, you can see the Arab villages and Jewish settlements scattered across the West Bank. Large Palestinian towns like Hebron, Jericho, and Ramallah are within easy commuting distance, and were it not for the conflict they surely would be well-developed suburbs solidly linked economically to Jerusalem. On my days off I sometimes drive southeast to the Dead Sea to hike among the canyons, and I am always amazed at how rapidly the stone and asphalt of Jerusalem melt away into the low rolling hills of the Judean desert. Just a few minutes after passing out of the easternmost neighborhoods of Jerusalem I find myself looking at Jordan on the horizon, with Jericho spilling out across the valley floor in front of me. It is here that Joshua led the Israelites across the Jordan River to settle the land, here that Jesus was baptized and spent forty days being tempted by Satan. Though the change in landscape is stark, I am barely aware that I am also passing into a different political zone. Because of the Israeli license plate on my car, I roll through the military checkpoints without being stopped, waved through by young soldiers who hardly give me a second glance. But for our patients living on the other side of the Green Line, making a journey of even just a mile or two between a West Bank town and Jerusalem can take hours, and may require long waits and searches. Palestinian patients often arrive late for appointments because of delays at the checkpoints. At the hospital, they frequently become anxious by midafternoon, pressing us to hurry up and finish whatever we have to do so that they can leave with enough time to make it home before nightfall, never knowing how long the crossing back into PA territory will take. On several occasions I have become alarmed by a Palestinian child who is drowsy and unresponsive during a clinic visit, as these are possible signs of infection or tumor progression. My alarm is replaced by embarrassed discomfort when the parent assures me that the child is fine, just exhausted from being awakened in the middle of the night in order to make it to the clinic in the morning.

At the end of the day, my colleagues and I often find ourselves, at the request of parents, admitting Palestinian patients for the night who could theoretically go home. Who can blame them for not wanting to subject a child who has just received hours of chemotherapy to standing for hours in a line at an outdoor checkpoint on a cold winter evening? What will they do if he starts to feel sick or to vomit, or starts shaking with the chills? My entire care management algorithm changes to adapt to the geopolitical situation. Children on chemotherapy who have low white blood cell counts are ordinarily sent home with the understanding that if they start to run a fever or feel sick, their parents will (hopefully) bring them right back. But while this may be easy for people living in Jerusalem and the surrounding Israeli towns, when the patients live in the West Bank I worry more. What happens if they arrive at a checkpoint during the night and can't get through quickly enough? What if the parents are afraid to travel after dark, afraid of encountering Israeli soldiers or Palestinian policemen on a mission? My calculations regarding when it is safe to send a child home suddenly become much more complex.

Like many Israelis, I feel conflicted about the military checkpoints, not to mention the "separation barrier" that wends its way across the hills. Having lived in Israel during the terrorist bombing campaigns of the 1990s, I am familiar with the constant anxiety of living under the threat of violence, how an unremarkable day spent running errands or meeting friends for coffee can without warning be transformed into a scene of horror. Like everyone else, I want everything possible to be done to prevent a return to those terrible times. But as a human being, as a Zionist, as someone who has come to Israel with a dream of what the place could be, the wall is a painful reminder of how far away peace can feel, how intense the hatred can be. When I treat my Palestinian patients I try not to think too much about what these sick children have to go through to get here and what they will have to endure to get home. I am living a privileged life in which I can avoid thinking about that sort of thing if I want to. But as I drive back to Tel Aviv in the evening and think about going for a jog by the sea or out with friends for a beer, I find myself wondering if my patients are still standing at a checkpoint, waiting to get home.

I am initially surprised at the number of Palestinians who come to Hadassah for treatment. I am also pleased. It's my hope that positive interactions between Israelis and Palestinians in a cancer clinic will lead to greater understanding and communi-

cation in non-healthcare settings as well. I'm also fascinated by
the idea of getting to know a people who are so close to me
geographically but who feel so far away politically and culturally. I know that health services in the PA are not as developed
as they are in Israel, and that children with cancer need the kind
of specialist care that is unavailable there. But I had assumed
that most Palestinian parents would seek medical care for their
children in Jordan or Egypt. Some do, but significant numbers of
Palestinians bring their children to Hadassah as well as to other
medical centers across Israel.

The process by which these children come to be under
our care remains somewhat opaque to me; it's nothing like the
straightforward referrals we get from community clinics in Israel.
Israeli children with a suspicion of cancer receive a referral form
filled out by their pediatrician and an appointment in our clinic
in a matter of days, if not hours. The pediatrician making the
referral can pick up the phone and call any of us in the department to arrange for an urgent consultation. And the national
healthcare system pays for it all. But when a Palestinian child is
diagnosed with cancer, a physician there must first write a letter
to our department requesting a consultation. Simply calling us to
discuss the patient is not an option. Once we have evaluated the
case and agreed to accept the child, the family must then obtain
a written financial guarantee from the PA Ministry of Health; it's
essentially a voucher that promises to cover the child's medical
expenses in Israel. Our billing department bills the PA for our
services the same way that they bill Israel's Ministry of Health,
and at the same rate. Palestinian parents hint to us that just getting the initial consultation letter, not to mention the financial
guarantee, is heavily dependent on personal connections, and
often even on bribes. Even worse, the financial guarantees are
doled out in amounts that cover only a limited number of treatments, so in order to cover the entire cost of therapy the families
must periodically return to the PA to repeat the approval process

again and again. With rare exceptions, this all unfolds without my actually communicating directly with anyone in the PA. Once treatment is under way, I periodically fill out a standardized form for each Palestinian child, requesting another allotment of funds for upcoming visits. I hand the form to the family, and then it is up to them to bring it to the Palestinian authorities.

There are other, more significant and uncomfortable, differences between how Israeli and Palestinian children get treated at Hadassah. When a European pharmaceutical company introduces a new drug, one whose impact on the treatment of a rare cancer is still unclear and that may increase the chance of survival by only a few percentage points, the question arises as to whether that drug should be included in what's known as "the basket," the list of drugs covered by Israel's national health insurance. What if the drug costs a quarter of a million dollars for one course of treatment? How do you decide the dollar value of a few additional percentage points in calculating a child's chance for survival? Sometimes the Israeli health ministry decides that because the drug in question has been incorporated into European cancer trials, the government will also cover the cost for Israeli children to get it. But the PA, facing more difficult financial constraints, may point to the fact that the Food and Drug Administration in the United States has not approved the drug and decide that therefore they will not cover the cost of the drug for Palestinian children. So we are left in the strange position of having some patients under our care who are receiving this particular medication and some who are not. And, of course, all of the parents talk to one another—even Israelis and Palestinians. So I find myself in one room explaining to a Palestinian family why they really shouldn't worry that their child isn't receiving this drug, because it has no proven effect and it isn't part of the standard of care, and then a moment later in another room explaining to an Israeli family why they should tolerate the many additional weeks of treatment involved with the administration of the drug, not to mention the risk of side effects such as chills and fever that may come with it. It's an uncomfortable situation, but there's really nothing I can do about it. Though our hospital is located in Israel, we are effectively working in two parallel healthcare systems.

PALESTINIANS NEED SPECIAL PASSES to enter Israel, especially if they will be staying for several days. This includes not only our patients but also the relatives who accompany them to Hadassah for their treatments. Sometimes, one of these relatives—occasionally even a parent—is not granted a pass. When I ask other staff members about this, the response is always a veiled suggestion that the individual denied permission must be on some sort of watch list, with the implication that it is most likely for terrorist activities. Once in a while, family members of a patient approach me, asking that I write a letter to push for a relative to be allowed entry into Israel. There's a woman at Hadassah whose job it is to liaise with both the PA and Israeli security forces, and I am told to turn these requests over to her, which I do, grateful that I don't have to wade into the middle of something I clearly don't understand. What if I help someone get in, ostensibly to visit a sick nephew, and he ends up committing an act of terrorism, maybe even killing someone? The parents whom I refer to the liaison know why I'm doing this; most likely all they want is to allow an uncle to see his nephew one last time before he dies. It always makes me feel terrible. I want to believe that illness and medicine transcend politics. I want to act as an impartial healer. But sometimes I just can't; this is the reality we live with here.

Because Hamas has been governing Gaza since 2007, it's almost impossible for Palestinians there to get their children to Hadassah for treatment. There's a procedure in place that allows Gazan Palestinians into Israel, but I'm sure it's even more complicated and time consuming than getting through the checkpoints in the West Bank. How the few Gazan Palestinians that come to us for treatment get here isn't something I fully understand. I just know that it's quite a testimony to the resourcefulness and resolve of parents trying to get the best care possible for their children.

I HAVE BEEN WAITING ALL DAY to see a new consult, a little boy we have been told will be coming from Gaza for evaluation of a new mass. By the end of the day we haven't heard anything from the family, so I assume that their plans changed and that they either went to a different hospital or decided the checkpoints were just too much to endure. Just as I'm leaving for home in the early evening, I pass an Arab woman walking into the lobby with a little boy trotting along behind her. Something about her makes me pause; the clinics in the building are all closed for the day, but she has the distinctly determined and slightly harried look of a parent trying to get her child to a late appointment. Using a passing colleague as an interpreter, I ask if I can help, figuring she must be looking for the emergency room. But no, it turns out this is the very child I had been waiting for all day. With our clinic closed until the morning, there's nothing I can do for them now. I call Mickey to confer with him. We're in a bit of a bind. I can't ask this woman and her child to travel all the way back to Gaza and return first thing in the morning. But I also technically can't admit him to our department as an inpatient because their paperwork permits only a daytime clinic visit. We agree that I will help them make up a bed in a corner of the lounge area and that I will try to beg a couple of meal trays from the evening food service. The whole situation is incredibly frustrating, both because I wish I could do better for this family right now, and more selfishly because I'm exhausted after a long day at work that has just gotten even longer. I find myself snapping at the mother, who just stares back at me expressionless, which makes me feel even worse. I call Mickey to vent my guilt and my frustration.

"Dr. Waldman," he says, and I can hear the laughter, and maybe some sadness, in his voice. "Do you really think that you are the biggest obstacle that this woman has had to overcome today? She's made it across multiple military checkpoints, through Hamas militants and the Israeli army, and traveled miles on roads she doesn't know just to get here. And you think that your annoyance is going to ruin her day? Save your coronaries, let the staff make her a bed, and you go home."

As I get to know more Palestinian patients from the West Bank, I also begin to learn its geography better, slowly becoming familiar with the names of small Arab villages and towns. Abeer is a nine-year-old girl from a village near Jericho. Looking like any other kid, she's wearing jeans and a T-shirt the first time she comes in to see us, the only difference being that she has a pronounced limp and, because of a large tumor protruding from her ankle, she's wearing only one shoe. Though at first shy, Abeer eventually warms to our staff when her treatment begins, especially once we manage to provide some pain relief. And although we have to communicate with Abeer through an interpreter, I am amazed at how much can be accomplished with my few words of broken Arabic (which, like my Hebrew, no doubt sounds hilarious in my clumsy American accent) and some friendly gestures. I soon feel that we have a warm, if largely nonverbal, relationship.

I try my best to develop some basic Arabic language skills, building off of an intensive summer course I had taken in college. I want my Arab-speaking patients and their families to feel that I'm at least trying to meet them halfway. I often wonder what Palestinians are thinking when they first arrive for treatment at Hadassah, what they make of our department, our staff, me. What have their past experiences with Israelis been, and with what preconceived notions do they arrive? Do they see me, an

American Jew, as yet another occupier, a foreign transplant who has come to take their land? Or do they view me, as I hope they do, in a comforting, hopeful light—as someone who has come to this place because I want to be able to help their children when they get sick? With my attempts to show kindness to these kids, to learn their language, I hope that I represent to them a more compassionate, more liberal side of the Zionist enterprise. Although I'm curious to know, I resist the impulse to flat-out ask them, in part to preserve the doctor-patient relationship and in part out of fear of the answers I might get.

Abeer arrives for each appointment accompanied only by her mother. Though we encourage—even insist—that both parents be present for at least the initial conversations regarding the diagnosis and treatment of a new patient, Abeer's father has never shown up. We eventually discover that this is because he is in a Palestinian jail. I don't ask the obvious question. I'm not sure I really want to know the answer to this question, either.

Abeer is fortunate, in the perverse way that we are able to talk about children with cancer having any luck at all. It's always seemed slightly nauseating to me when someone says that a child has a "good" form of cancer, as if such a thing could truly exist. I understand the sentiment, but the bottom line is that the only "good" cancer to have is no cancer. Nevertheless, the good news in Abeer's case is that her tumor, a Ewing's sarcoma, usually responds well to chemotherapy. The initial screening studies show no sign of metastasis, so her chance of being cured is fairly good—about 70 percent of children with Ewing's sarcoma do not experience a recurrence. "Good news" is, of course, relative. Would you be pleased if your child had a 70 percent chance of being cured? What if you were told she had a 30 percent chance of dying? Statistics in oncology, as anywhere else, can be slippery; in the end, a 99 percent cure rate is meaningless when your child is the other 1 percent.

The less fortunate aspect of Abeer's situation is that in the months that it took to navigate the bureaucracy necessary to get her from her village to our department for her treatments, the mass has grown to engulf her entire ankle. From the very first appointment we hint to Abeer's mother that there is a good chance that the only way we will be able to achieve local eradication of the disease will be by amputating Abeer's leg below the knee. Though theoretically radiation might be used in place of surgery for this type of tumor, because of the tumor's location and size this would probably leave her ankle a hardened mass of fibrosis and scarring, rendering her severely disabled. Amputation would offer the advantage (again, such a strange term to be used in the context of such horrors) of both ensuring that the mass is completely removed and allowing for the fitting of a prosthetic leg, which would enable Abeer to have a better physical, functional, and psychological recovery.

After several courses of chemotherapy the tumor is much smaller, but it's just not small enough for us to simply excise it. The surgeons will have to amputate the leg. Abeer's mother is, unsurprisingly, devastated, though we try to emphasize that amputation will likely lead to a better overall outcome. Much as it was with Lena's family, the grief here feels like something deeper than just sadness over a daughter's impending disfigurement. I feel the culture gap, sense that there is some space that I am failing to bridge, a wound I can't address because I can't yet define it. Abeer's mother expresses concern about what amputation will mean for her daughter's future social status, her ability to get married, to fit into society. It is as though she fears the amputation will actually change Abeer's value as a person. And, of course, I am not a parent, much less a mother, so there is a dimension to her anguish that eludes me.

The chief nurse in our outpatient clinic is a woman named Fatma, an Israeli Arab who has devoted her entire career to Hadassah. Through Fatma, I ask for permission to speak directly with Abeer about the prospect of amputation. After some hesitation her mother agrees, because by this time she has developed some trust in us. We sit in a small office, the four of us, and settle into what is now for me the increasingly familiar and strangely comforting rhythm of a difficult conversation conducted via translation. We proceed phrase by phrase: me in Hebrew to Fatma, Fatma in Arabic to Abeer, Abeer in Arabic back to her, Fatma in Hebrew back to me, all conveyed slowly and in low tones. Fatma has told me in the past that she can sense when I am preparing to convey difficult news because my voice becomes lower and my tone softens. Knowing that I can be hot-tempered outside of work, she jokes that I should try this more often outside the hospital as well.

We explain things carefully to Abeer, showing her the X-rays of her leg, as well as images on a computer that help illustrate what a prosthesis looks like. We emphasize that the goal is to cure her, and that we hope that after the surgery and some more chemotherapy she will be healthy for the rest of her life. She is stoic at first, and even asks a few good questions. But at a certain point she falls apart, weeping, and the discussion lapses into silence, the rhythm broken. Abeer's mother sits by her side, also quietly crying. Fatma takes over, leaning in close, quietly murmuring to Abeer, not bothering to stop and translate for me. After a few minutes Fatma looks over at me and says, "Okay, enough for now."

"Where are we?" I ask, having lost my place in the conversation.

"It's okay," she repeats, "just let them go home and come back next week. It will be okay."

Whether she has been speaking in a way that is culturally coded to better connect with Abeer and her mother or as only someone who is herself a mother would be able to, I do not know. But I trust Fatma completely, and even though I don't know exactly how matters stand, I relinquish control of this situation to her and wrap up the conversation.

At the next clinic visit a week later Abeer is much calmer, and she displays a steely determination to continue the discussion. She begins by stating that she understands that the amputation is going to happen, and then she asks specific questions about what she will and won't be able to do afterward, in particular whether she will be able to dance. I am in awe of her maturity and amazed at how a nine-year-old is able, after such a short time, to proclaim that she is ready for a life-changing surgery. Her mother interjects with just one last request, that we give her a chance to confer with Abeer's father. It's a bit embarrassing to be reminded that there is another important figure in this story whose existence I seem to have forgotten. Of course he should be updated, and I should have thought to mention it myself. We send them off and I assume that when they return for Abeer's next appointment we can begin discussing with them the preparations for the surgery. So it comes as a shock when Abeer's mother informs us that we cannot go ahead with the surgery because her husband won't allow it.

"Doesn't he realize her life is at stake?" I ask.

"Yes," she says, "he realizes. But he would rather not have a daughter at all than have one who is damaged. She must keep her foot at all costs."

Fatma and I confer, and I am relieved to see that she, too, seems appalled by the turn of events. We decide that the best thing would be for us to speak directly with Abeer's father. Because it's illegal and not altogether safe for Israeli citizens to enter PA-administered territory, a personal visit to see him in jail is out of the question. We ask the social worker assigned to Abeer, also an Israeli Arab, to coordinate a telephone conference call. This turns out to be a far more complicated task than I had thought, though for reasons that I can't completely decipher. Communication seems to fail at multiple levels. The social worker keeps trying to connect with the appropriate authorities in the prison, but they do not seem inclined to help us. And even if I do get to have a conversation with Abeer's father, I'm not sure how I will manage to convey my concerns in one brief phone call to a man with whom I could not have less in common. There doesn't seem to be any prison official, physician, or social worker on the other side whom we can call for help. I am at a loss.

I have run into this before when dealing with Palestinian patients. Back in the United States, when one of my patients would be admitted to another medical center with an emergency, the first thing that the clinicians there would do would be to call me to coordinate care. Here in Israel, with rare exceptions, when my Palestinian patients go back home to Gaza or to the West Bank, it feels like they are disappearing into a black hole. I never get a single phone call from a Palestinian clinician. Perhaps I'm being naive, but it's hard for me to understand how medical professionals allow regional politics to get in the way of taking care of children who are being treated for cancer. I hear several theories on this subject from colleagues. I am told that the families of our patients try to obscure the fact that they are receiving care in Israel, that there is something shameful and unpatriotic about it. I am told that they fear reprisal for having sought help from the Zionist enemy, that if they do have to go to an emergency room in the PA, they may be treated less well. And I am told that Palestinian clinicians won't reach out to us for advice and coordination of care due to fear, anger, or disdain. And so that is why we have reached this point, where the key player in deciding Abeer's fate, her father, is just a faceless, voiceless entity lost in a system that is inaccessible to me.

Eventually, and after much effort, the social worker does manage to orchestrate a telephone conversation with Abeer's father, but the breakthrough happens so suddenly and unexpectedly that I am not present to participate. The social worker, who is familiar with the details of the treatment plan, reports back to me that despite all of her explanations, Abeer's father is unwilling to consent to the amputation. The conversation goes nowhere. I can't help but wonder if the outcome would have been different if we'd had an ongoing, personal relationship with him, if the Israeli doctor who wants to cut off his daughter's leg was more than a faceless, voiceless entity on the other side of the separation wall. But maybe it wouldn't have. Maybe Abeer's father really would rather have a dead daughter than a daughter without a leg. Hard as that is for me to imagine, I'll never know.

With amputation not an option, I seek the second-best solution. We decide to proceed with a course of radiation therapy, hoping that it will kill any active tumor cells. If it works, we would then send Abeer for rehabilitation. Hopefully this will eliminate or reduce the fibrosis and allow her to regain partial use of her leg. I try to explain this to Abeer and her mother in a positive, upbeat way, but I am once again dogged by the feeling that I have failed my patient. What if the radiation doesn't completely eliminate the cancer and Abeer dies? Will it be because I didn't do my job properly? Or would this simply have been a case of my having no option but to bow to forces beyond my control?

Though we like to think of oncology as a science—a combination of studies, statistics, drugs, and dosages—so much of what oncologists do actually depends on the art of effective communication. And it is there that we so often fail. When I was working in the United States, even though I was just starting out I already had a sense that our medical community often seemed to fall short in our efforts to communicate effectively with our patients. One reason often given is the time constraints placed on a busy practice. Another, more fundamental, reason is the lack of instruction in communication skills during medical training. Even in the training to be an oncologist, where difficult conversations are a daily occurrence, there was scant attention paid to advanced communication skills and few opportunities even to observe more senior colleagues demonstrating their skills. What I am finding here in Israel is that the additional factors of multiple cultural and religious traditions, the incendiary politics of the area, and language differences can make effective communication seem almost impossible. Even within the hospital, in my day-to-day work, I struggle to decipher the code of conduct among a staff composed of a motley crew of immigrants and natives. I love the fact that here at Hadassah we are Israeli Arabs, Israeli Jews, immigrants from all over the world, religious and secular, each with his or her own sense of proper behavior and appropriate interactions. But my training in New York has not prepared me for how to conduct discussions with my colleagues, many of whom have styles and manners much different from my own. In the United States, even with all of the diversity among patients and clinicians, the tendency is for everyone to try to adhere to a standard, albeit somewhat bland, model of conduct in the hospital. That doesn't mean that communication is so successful, just that there is more of a system-wide uniformity in how people conduct themselves. Everyone is polite, patient, even solicitous. Here in Israel that model doesn't appear to exist. The same things that make the country so appealing to me—the proud expressions of diversity, the de-emphasis on personal space, the overfamiliarity to the point of rudeness—become a double-edged sword. On the one hand it engenders a sense of family and inclusiveness. On the other hand, in the workplace, where I am still learning how to navigate communication with patients and colleagues alike, the often unpredictable nature of people's behavior makes it difficult for me to understand the rules of conduct. Potential barriers to communication abound, whether it's different ideas about religion, different cultural traditions, or a concrete barrier that's been put up by my government to keep us safe. I have come here with the specific intention of integrating with people in a setting very different from the one I trained in. I am only just beginning to recognize how truly difficult this is going to be, even with the best and most noble of intentions.

4

Silence

SARA IS A UNIVERSITY STUDENT in her early twenties with a recurrence of a rare connective tissue tumor. When she was first diagnosed a few years ago, her parents had initially sought treatment for her at a medical center in America, driven by the belief that this is where one goes for the gold standard in cancer treatment. Here at Hadassah I have become accustomed to parents asking me, during the initial workup phase, whether there are better treatments available for their child abroad that they should explore. Or whether there are better, more expensive drugs available here in Israel that they aren't getting because it's not included in the national insurance basket.

"Doctor," they will say, leaning in conspiratorially, "between us, is there anywhere else we should go? We have private insurance, you know. Money is not an issue."

Knowing that I come from a well-known cancer center in the United States, they ask whether they should go there. Or, better yet, why don't I just call up my former colleagues and get instructions from them on how to provide care, saving the family the trip abroad? I understand their desire to do everything they possibly can for their sick child, but I am irritated by the implication that I have one set of recommendations for families with money and another set for families without.

"I promise," I respond, "that if I know of a better treatment anywhere—in the United States, in Europe, in the mountains of Tibet—I will send you there."

In reality, most first-line cancer therapies for children in Israel are exactly the same as those offered in Europe and North America, because most Israeli pediatric oncologists participate in or at least use protocols that are generated by international consortia. The real difference that I find between Israel and the United States in terms of cancer treatments is the relative dearth of formal clinical trials available for children in Israel with recurrent or progressive disease. The United States and Western Europe are the places to go for that type of treatment. Of course, by the time a child gets to that point, the odds of his being cured are usually pretty poor, so whether to travel abroad for an experimental drug trial or to remain in Israel for some cobbled-together protocol becomes a difficult decision. Many families don't realize that phase-one drug trials are designed primarily to study what dose of a drug is even safe for use in humans. The odds that a drug in a phase-one trial might help are actually lower than the odds that the drug may hurt or even kill a patient. Still, many cling to the hope that they will win the cancer lottery and that their child will be that rare one who enters a trial and gets a drug that turns out to be a cure.

"My child already defied the odds by getting cancer, which is rare as well," they often say, with a heartbreakingly convoluted logic. "Why shouldn't they beat the odds again and also be the one who responds to a new treatment?"

But for the most part, though they almost always ask, when it comes to front-line therapies very few Israeli families feel the need to seek treatment abroad. Sara, who has come to Hadassah for treatment because her tumor has recurred, has reversed the usual process. Her parents, aware of the near certainty of a poor outcome, allow Sara to assert herself as an independent young adult and to make her own decisions. Though her mother often accompanies her to appointments, she remains for the most part quietly in the background. And Sara, who is no longer a child, has asked me not to speak with her parents in her absence. Though she tells me that she feels close with her parents, she says that there are certain things she prefers not to discuss with them.

Hospitals have varying policies on how to determine which patients should be treated by pediatric oncologists and which by adult oncologists. Some have a firm policy of sending all patients over the age of eighteen or twenty-one to the adult oncologists, while others are more flexible and take into consideration the type of cancer the patient has. Though she's in her early twenties, because the type of tumor Sara has is more typically found in children, we agree to treat her in our department. In fact, there is increasing data to support this approach, and a number of studies over the past decade or so have suggested that adolescents and young adults with pediatric-type tumors fare better when treated according to pediatric protocols. Our department better suits Sara's personality as well. She's a bright young woman, studying for a degree in philosophy, but there is nonetheless something childlike about her. At times while she's talking to one of us, or even just sitting quietly, she displays a flash of unexpected fragility or a brief outburst of petulance. Some of the staff label this as regression, but to me that seems unfair; at her age she may be legally an adult, but when has that ever precisely correlated with emotional or developmental age?

As time goes by, my roster of patients at Hadassah includes more and more children with a low likelihood of cure. This is in part a function of the fact that, though most children with sarcomas have a relatively good chance of cure, those with metastatic disease at diagnosis or who experience a relapse do much worse. But on a more fundamental level I am drawn to the care of these particular children because it speaks to my ongoing interest in theology and the humanities. I am fascinated by how patients and families respond to the challenges of life-threatening illness, some seeming to gather limitless strength while others seem to crumble. I'm curious about how I, as a clinician and a human being, should respond to families exposed to this sort of suffering, something I was never taught during my training. And, of course, I'm still trying to figure out how it all fits into my own values and beliefs.

Though Mickey and I share Sara's care, she is often scheduled for appointments on my clinic days. I enjoy my interactions with her. Sara is an interesting, thoughtful young woman, and I like hearing about her studies, which resonate with my own interest in theology. Once the clinic has quieted down in the afternoon, I will often take a break from my charts and sit with her to chat about philosophy while she's getting her chemotherapy infusions. As the tumor gradually progresses despite the treatments, Sara starts to speak more specifically about her own existential concerns. I just listen, trying to read between the lines to glean any information that might be clinically relevant, anything that might help guide our decision making regarding her treatment. I think of the patient's father who once joked that I was now doing applied theology; Sara, faced with her own mortality, might similarly be said to be doing applied philosophy.

Sara's disease progresses slowly. I want to believe this is due to the "tailored" treatments she is receiving from us, but now that I have a bit more experience in oncology, I am no longer convinced of how much control we actually exert over anything. Despite our best efforts, tumors often grow, regress, or stall in ways that don't obviously correlate with our interventions. Sara's disease, mostly in her lungs now, grows slowly enough so that she has plenty of time to be aware that it's happening. She notices as the weeks pass that her cough is getting worse, that more often than not she has to sleep propped up by pillows, using gravity to help keep her airways open. Our interactions, both during the morning clinic visits and during our informal afternoon philosophy sessions, begin to involve more quiet sitting than talking. When she does speak, Sara requires longer pauses to catch her breath and to compose her thoughts. In the gaps between sentences we listen to the wet crackles of her congested lungs. She becomes angrier and more fearful, and she pours her dwindling energy into explosive philosophical outbursts: on whether or not God exists, what we are actually here for, what it all means. I don't share with her my own thoughts and doubts about these questions. I mostly just listen and reflect. The silence between these outbursts, the negative space of the quiet interludes, takes on a substance of its own. In her unfinished or unspoken thoughts, I hear the things she cannot or will not say. Meaning is conveyed through silence.

Rabbi Heschel wrote of this sort of ineffable questioning of things that can't be articulated. "The mind does not know how to phrase it," he says, "yet the soul sighs it, sings it, pleads it." That there are no words to capture these thoughts does not make them less meaningful; their very inexpressibility speaks to their importance. Medicine is full of these numinous moments of awe. I caught glimpses of them as a trainee, but I am more attuned to them now. As I sit with Sara, I think back to the many long nights when I was in training in New York, where in keeping with our upside-down medical system the least trained clinician was left in charge of departments full of the sickest children. If I was lucky, relative quiet would descend on the wards by midnight. I would walk the halls quietly, pausing at each doorway to listen to the sounds of the children breathing in each bed, amazed and terrified that I had been given responsibility over them for the night. In my scrubs and sneakers I felt like a kid in pajamas, staying up late after the grown-ups had all gone out. I would scan my notes, scribbled earlier at evening sign-out, and review each child's condition, mentally checking off what I needed to worry about for the rest of the night, what I might be called on to do in an emergency. In the silence of the dimmed hospital hallway, I was achingly aware of the city around us, the people who might be getting ready for bed, or already sleeping, or out partying, while here in these halls we watched over these children and their families living out their own quiet dramas. Each bed contained its own story, and we were given the gift of playing a part—hopefully a useful part—in that story. I sensed even then that in that silence something like a sacred duty was to be found, that somewhere in there was the still, small voice in the whirlwind.

ONE DAY SARA ASKS TO MEET with both Mickey and me. We sit in a clinic room, door closed, listening to her rapid shallow breaths as she works herself up to saying something. Her cheeks and temples are sunken by this point, outward manifestations of the tumor inside that is ravenously consuming her. Her lips have become thin and pale, drawn back over now prominent teeth, and her eye sockets are sharply defined now that the surrounding fat has melted away. It is painfully obvious that Sara has the skeletal look of someone who is very ill and will soon die. Her words come in bursts, broken by dyspnea and by emotion.

"I'm getting worse," she states. "When I get to a certain point . . . I want you to promise . . . you will help me—"

We wait for her to finish the thought. Help with what? Beneath the sound of her breathing I can hear my own heartbeat, and in my head I run through different ways she might fill in that blank.

"I don't want to suffer . . . when it's time . . . help me finish."

The air around us feels heavy, those silent gaps now dreadfully dense with new meaning. Sara wants to know that we will help end her life when she feels it is time.

Mickey and I exchange glances, carefully thinking how best to reply. After a long pause she looks down. "Never mind . . . never mind," she says softly.

How terrible it must be for Sara to have these sorts of thoughts pent up inside her, swirling around in her head as she lies alone in the dark at night. And how hard it must be for her to give voice to them in the light of day, even to those she loves and trusts. We reassure her that we won't let her suffer, though we're careful to be clear that we will not actively hasten her death, which is of course illegal. But we promise that we won't abandon her. I've heard these sorts of fears expressed by patients before. The most common worry that I hear from children facing the possibility of death isn't actually that they will die. It is that when the time comes they will be alone, and that it will hurt. Those are two concerns we can take care of, and so we try to address them in replying to Sara. She barely responds, having retreated again into her own thoughts.

This conversation repeats itself two or three more times over the next few weeks, always a tearful plea followed quickly by a retraction, as though she is still testing the waters. Throughout, she continues to decline. As she grows weaker, requiring more and more medicine for pain and for shortness of breath, she is admitted to the hospital for better symptom management. Escalating doses of medicine that are needed for her comfort, combined with the effects of the progressing tumor, begin to make her more and more sleepy. One otherwise unremarkable morning she whispers to me that she is ready to sleep. Despite her frailty she is able to express herself enough that I understand what she means. She isn't asking me to do anything to hasten her death, or even to sedate her. She is simply and quietly stating that she is going to sleep. Saying goodbye. Her family gathers around the bed and she speaks with them for a while in hushed tones. I can't make out what she's saying, but it's not intended for me, anyway. For the next few days she appears to peacefully sleep, and we don't have to significantly adjust any of her medications. At this point the dying process has taken over, and her body has begun to shut down. Normally our bodies get rid of waste products through several organs: kidneys, liver, lungs. Now, with those organs failing one after another, like slowly falling dominoes, the rising levels of toxins in her body act as a sort of natural anesthetic, inducing a deeper and deeper slumber. The room is largely silent for those last few days, with just the whirring and beeping of our machines and the low murmurs of Sara's family whispering to her. Despite the silence, or perhaps because of it, there is a sense that so much more is happening.

ISRAEL OFTEN SEEMS TO RUN at full volume. So I learn to value the quieter moments, at work and during my free time, when I can indulge in reverie and introspection. I live in Neve Tzedek, an old neighborhood in the southwest part of Tel Aviv that, despite significant gentrification over the past few years, still retains the flavor of a village. My apartment is on the top floor of a narrow three-story building. Because of the slope of the neighborhood, I have a clear view across the rooftops to the nearby Mediterranean Sea. At night I can lie in bed and, if the wind is blowing just right, I can hear the sound of waves breaking on the shore. I often wake in the early morning darkness to the eerie and beautiful wailing of the muezzin from the mosques in nearby Jaffa, a sound that is at the same time foreign and comfortingly familiar. For the first few months, the muezzin has competition from a crowing rooster in a neighbor's yard, which lends a rustic charm to the proceedings, but then local stray cats put an end to him. The mournful cries of the muezzin continue to fill the air on their own.

There are of course other sounds in Israel that don't have quite the same soulful resonance. The sounds of the crowded Jerusalem city streets during the day—car horns honking, people yelling—are nothing more than unpleasant noise. For a country where human communication with God can often manifest itself in such sonorous, beautiful tones, the sounds of daily street life can seem terribly disharmonious, and even cruel. And while I enjoy the sense of being surrounded by history during my daily Tel Aviv–to–Jerusalem commute, my reverie is often interrupted by the madness of Israeli drivers. I look up into my rearview mirror to find cars tailing me at high speed within what seems like inches of my rear bumper, aggressively honking, weaving through impossibly narrow gaps in the traffic without signaling, slowing down, or even paying attention to what they are doing. Arriving safely at work and without losing my cool sometimes feels like a major accomplishment in itself.

THERE IS INDEED, as Ecclesiastes tells us, a time to be silent and a time to speak. In medicine, as in much of life, the trick is to figure out which is which—to know when to break the silence with an encouraging word or an empathetic murmur and, perhaps even more challenging, to know when to sit in silence and just be present. At Hadassah, our meetings with patients and families usually occur in the clinic examination rooms, where behind closed doors some degree of quiet and control can be maintained. But outside the rooms, in the hallway and treatment areas, a barely controlled chaos rules throughout the day. Things start out quietly in the morning. When patients arrive they check in with the triage nurse who sits alongside the exam rooms. They are then directed to one of the patient bays, where another nurse checks vital signs, accesses ports if necessary, and sends off blood tests to the lab. Patients and their families then wait their turn to be called to an exam room to be seen by a doctor. Once a patient is seen, she returns to the treatment area, where a nurse proceeds according to the doctor's orders—starting chemotherapy, administering other medications or fluids, or simply discharging the patient for the day. Questions come up. Nurses thread their way through the increasingly clogged hallway between the treatment area and the exam rooms, double-checking orders, notifying doctors of changes, ensuring that the machinery of the clinic keeps running. As the day progresses, personal space evaporates. By noon there is a din of laughter, crying, yelling, blaring televisions, and videogames. The crowd alongside the exam rooms swells, creating a logjam at the clinic entrance, with parents pressing the overwhelmed triage nurse to try to get their child in next, to make sure he has not been forgotten. The clinic becomes a heaving mass, with staff trying to maintain some semblance of order over it all. It's very different from anything I experienced at hospitals back in the United States, which always felt to me more organized but also less warm, more impersonal. At first I delight in the clamor. It tickles some Zionist nerve in my subconscious. It's like we're all one big family, and the pushiness and lack of respect for personal boundaries, so often interpreted by outsiders as rudeness, just means we all feel comfortable and close to one another. But after a while it begins to grate on me. There are enough elements in pediatric oncology that are chaotic and beyond my control as it is, and allowing the clinic environment to become even a little bit unruly quickly becomes more anxiety-provoking than charming or familial. I've never been much of a type-A perfectionist, but relative to what goes on some days in the clinic, at times I feel like a drill sergeant in my desire for precision and order. A recurrent point of contention is different cultural interpretations of what a closed exam room door means. When I sit in an exam room with a patient and her family, the idea is to shut out all of the chaos of the clinic. We try to create a private space where nothing else in the world matters other than the delicate, carefully constructed conversation that is happening here and now. But when nurses barge in without knocking, looking for syringes or cotton balls or whatever in the supply cabinets, I quickly lose my cool. The disruption to the conversation taking place can completely undermine what I'm trying to accomplish. Even worse are interruptions when I am in the middle of a physical exam, when a patient lies exposed and vulnerable on the exam table. I try to explain this to the staff, but to no avail. I start locking the exam room door, which is clearly off-putting for the families in the room with me, as the sound of the sliding bolt has a definite "you're not getting out of here" tone. The door locking also deeply offends the nurses, who take it as an indication of a lack of trust. "But no matter how much I ask, people still just barge in without knocking," I protest. I receive assurances that are quickly forgotten. I briefly try putting a DO NOT DISTURB sign on the door if there is a difficult discussion going on, but that proves unworkable. How do you decide which conversations in a pediatric oncology clinic are the difficult ones?

THOUGH THE NATURE OF PEDIATRIC ONCOLOGY is fundamentally sad, we collectively make an effort to maintain an upbeat atmosphere in our department. As in many other pediatric oncology wards throughout the world, the walls are painted in bright colors and adorned with playful and festive decorations, images of cartoon characters, and friendly animals. There are activities like cooking classes, arts-and-crafts projects, and magic shows, and wonderful clowns who wander through the department to help brighten everyone's day. One mother tells me that a friend recently commented on how sad it must be for her six-year-old to have to come to the clinic almost daily. She laughs ruefully. People don't believe her when she says that her son loves coming here, that he looks forward to seeing his friends at the hospital. He actually had a temper tantrum one day when it turned out that he wouldn't get his planned chemotherapy due to low blood counts and would have to go right home instead of staying to play videogames with the other kids.

Volunteers who come to spend time with the children and

their families play an important part in maintaining the cheery atmosphere. The largest and best organized group consists of Orthodox Jewish teenage girls who, in lieu of regular military service, spend a year doing volunteer work in schools, hospitals, and children's homes to fulfill their national service requirement. Their work is incredibly important, though they have a tendency to get a bit carried away with their mission, at times bursting into the clinic singing at the tops of their lungs and clapping their hands, surging through our department like raging flood-waters. One afternoon I'm sitting with parents in a quiet room, talking through difficult news as they fight back tears, when we are distracted by raucous singing and laughter right outside the door. I excuse myself and go into the hallway to ask the volun-teers politely to keep it down and maybe move farther down the hall. They contain themselves for a few minutes but quickly start back up again. By the third time that I have to ask them to lower the volume, I can tell my tone is not at all polite and my body language more aggressive. I'm not sure if my openly expressed anger is a sign that I'm learning to fit in here, or if my annoyance at behavior that no one else seems to be bothered about is a sign that I'm not.

On another occasion, I'm on call on a Saturday evening and I telephone the nursing station to check in on a little boy in Room Eleven, which has been primarily designed for children who are approaching the end of life. It's just a bit bigger and more com-fortable than the other rooms, better able to accommodate fami-lies, and, with no window in the door, a bit more private as well.

On this particular evening, the occupant is a Palestinian boy, an eight-year-old with a progressive muscle tumor. We've been treating him for months as an outpatient, but now, with a tumor starting to compress his brainstem, it's become too much for his parents to handle his care at home. They've been here with him for days, holding a vigil at his bedside. Chanted verses from the Koran quietly fill the room from a phone plugged into the wall. I want to make sure that he's comfortable in what are likely his final hours. While I'm waiting for his nurse to come to the phone, I hear in the background what sounds like a crowd of people, accompanied by an acoustic guitar, loudly singing songs to welcome the new week now that the Jewish Sabbath has ended. When the nurse comes to the phone I ask about the noise, suggesting that it be kept down. They are volunteers, she says, entertaining some of the patients in the family area. Unfortunately, the family area happens to be inconveniently located right next to Room Eleven. The nurse is speaking to me from halfway down the hall, yet the singing is so loud that even if I put the phone down I can still make out the words. She says she has already told them that there is a very sick child in the next room but was basically ignored. I ask to speak with the leader of the group. Someone with an adult voice gets on, which infuriates me even further, since he should know better. I know that part of my anger is just my own stress reaction to caring for a dying patient. But part of it isn't; it's a reaction to unequivocal rudeness. I tell him that he has five minutes to get the volunteers out of the department. We cannot have this degree of singing and noise, I explain, no matter how well meaning, while a child is dying. It troubles me that this is something I would never have had to explain in a hospital in New York.

When I call the nursing station back ten minutes later, nothing has changed. If anything, the singing seems louder, although at this point it may just be that my anger is affecting my perception. The nurse reports that our patient appears to be either sleeping or unconscious, but I'm still concerned about his parents, trying to listen to the Koran on their speakerphone. I call Mickey, who sighs as he hears the anger in my voice; he has apparently had to deal with this before. He calls the head of the hospital, who in turn calls into the department and asks the group to move outside. Unfazed, they simply relocate to the downstairs lobby, from where they can still be heard five floors up, the noise now reverberating through the central atrium of the building. It is as though by not leaving, by maybe even increasing the volume of their singing, they think they are winning some sort of contest, though I'm not sure what they're trying to prove.

I feel a twinge of discomfort about the racial and religious component in this situation. I'm sure the volunteers have seen family members come and go from Room Eleven, so they know they are Arabs. It may be my imagination, but I often get the feeling that some of the religious volunteers seem just a little bit less concerned about what is going on in the rooms with Arab patients. This certainly isn't true of everyone, and Mickey projects a very clear message throughout the department that this is a place for all sick children, regardless of ethnicity, religion, or politics. But the occasional whiff of favoritism on the individual level is undeniable, and I can't help but notice which kids the volunteers spend most of their time with.

I MOVED TO ISRAEL SPECIFICALLY to live as a Jew in a Jewish state, and so I'm surprised by how uncomfortable I feel when I realize that while the hospital is always appropriately decked out for every Jewish holiday, Muslim and Christian holidays get barely a nod, at best a small display in a corner. The only way I learn about the Muslim holidays, the fasts and the feasts, is when patients ask if their treatment schedules can be adjusted to allow them to be at home with family for celebrations.

Fatma, the head nurse in our pediatric oncology clinic, soon becomes a dear friend. An Israeli Arab in her fifties who lives in an Arab neighborhood in West Jerusalem, she has risen through the ranks from staff nurse to head nurse. She enjoys a reputation as a respected member of the hospital community whose opinions on matters both medical and administrative are highly valued. But none of this exempts her from the identity politics of the region that, unfortunately, spill into our hospital at times, the whiff of racism and nationalist sentiment that I pick up on here and there. My Arabic is not good enough to understand her conversations with the Palestinian families of our patients, but Fatma tells me that they often treat her as though she is a traitor, an Arab Uncle Tom. My Hebrew, on the other hand, is quite good enough to pick up on the thinly veiled (and sometimes not veiled at all) racism with which some Israeli Jews treat her. One day, after I'd been at Hadassah more than a year, I'm in a new consultation with the family of a young boy with a connective tissue tumor. The parents are religious Jews from the United States who moved to Israel not long before I did and now live in a town just across the Green Line. We spend a few minutes establishing a rapport, sharing our experiences of making aliyah. In the middle of the discussion, Fatma knocks on the door, ducking into the room to get something from a cabinet. After taking a moment to warmly greet the family—in Hebrew—and welcome them to our department, she slips out again. As the door closes behind her, the father looks at me, leans forward, and, in a slightly lower tone of voice, asks, "So . . . is she okay?"

I stare at him, unsure what to say. Though he's speaking English, I'm still somehow hoping I've misunderstood.

"I mean," he continues, "is this safe? I have to be honest, I'm a little uncomfortable with an Arab being in charge of my son's care."

I want to vomit. Or to hit him. This is the opposite of everything I came to Israel for, everything I believe the state should be. And beyond my disgust at his racism is my anger at this insult to a cherished colleague and friend, a person with whom I spend so much time that the other nurses have started to refer to me jokingly as "Fatma's fifth child."

I want to let this man know in no uncertain terms how I feel. But his son is going to be my patient and I'm going to have to have a relationship with this family, so I have to be careful about what I say. I reassure him, telling him that I trust Fatma with my life and that she's one of the best nurses I've ever worked with, anywhere. I try to say it all in a manner that ignores the underlying implication of his statement: that Arabs can't be trusted, that they are inherently our enemies and out to get us. I tell myself that I'm just addressing the technical aspect of his question, whether his son is in competent hands. But I can't help but feel that I am betraying her, and myself, by not calling him out on his disgraceful question. This is what the Zionist dream has become: two American Israeli Jews sitting in Jerusalem, taking positions on the merits and trustworthiness of an Arab woman with roots in this city that go back centuries.

There are other incidents, some with sabras, native-born Israelis, and some with *olim,* new immigrants like myself. I feel anger at the sabras because they force me to acknowledge ugly aspects of a culture that is very different from what I had dreamed it would be, and at the *olim* because as fellow immigrants they embarrass me. One morning I'm confronted by a parent, an American Israeli like myself, who yells at me that his daughter, who has been admitted for chemotherapy, had to move out of her room in the middle of the night to make space for a Palestinian teenager being urgently admitted with a life-threatening infection. "Come on," he says, without a trace of shame, "I saw who got moved into that room." In one of the few instances where I actually confront a parent for this sort of behavior, I tell him that if I hear him speak that way again, we will transfer his child's care to another hospital of his choosing. The argument ends in a draw, each of us disgusted with the other. In large part as a result of Mickey's efforts these incidents are not common, but they occur just often enough to remind me how much incivility percolates just below the surface.

I FIND IT RATHER IRONIC that one thing all the cheerful and not-so-cheerful chaos in our department has taught me is the value and importance of silence. The goal of treatment is, of course, a cured patient in permanent remission. But the reality of our daily work revolves around much more complex, nuanced conversations. This needs to be done in a quiet, sheltering space. And sometimes an important element in this process is simply sitting with patients in silence, so they can process what we are telling them and not feel alone. As was the case with Sara, at times I feel I have constructed entire conversations around silence, as though the stillness in the room was somehow made solid, formed into the walls and beams that created the space around us.

John Cage famously created an architecture of time and space out of silence in his musical composition entitled *4'33"*. Like many people, when I first heard of this piece I thought it was a joke, some sort of obscure modernist pun. But after I'd been practicing medicine for a few years, it began to make more sense. When I listen to recordings of the piece (which I actually do now and then), I hear not just the silence but everything in between: a scraping chair, a cough, people shifting in their seats, my own breathing, my own heartbeat. And it all occurs in a precisely defined space of time, between the conductor's signal to start and the conclusion of the piece, so that there is indeed a sense of architecture, of planning. Though, of course, I never actually time the periods of silence while I sit with patients, as I evolve as a physician I become more aware of them. When I first began working with patients, these silences made me feel deeply uncomfortable. Even now, after years of practice, I still have to fight the urge to say something during these silences, to fill them with something, anything, though I now know how much is really going on in those spaces. I've learned the importance of simply sitting there, of just being present. More often than not, a patient will eventually articulate some critically important, at times even beautiful, statement or question that will set the course for the rest of the discussion. I now make it a point of intentionally incorporating periods of silence in my conversations with my patients and their families.

.   .   .

NOAM IS A FOUR-YEAR-OLD GIRL with a rare tumor of
the pancreas. I never really get to know her because by the time
she becomes my patient she is so sick that she is always either
sleeping in bed or lying listlessly in her parents' arms. When she
was initially diagnosed, the tumor had already grown so large
that it could not be surgically removed. Several courses of chemotherapy do nothing except make this thin, jaundiced girl feel
worse and grow even thinner and more jaundiced. In terms of
realistic treatment protocols, we quickly arrive at the end of the
line; there is no more tumor-directed therapy to offer. We have
tried to initiate conversations about the next steps, but her parents have been resistant, recognizing that the only thing really
left to discuss is how to navigate her death. There is a sense
of deadlock. Every time a staff member tries to bring this up,
Noam's parents shut the conversation down. I feel that I'm not
making any progress in my discussions with them in the clinic,
and so I am selfishly somewhat relieved when she is admitted to
the hospital because she is running a fever and needs nutritional
support. Now that Noam is an inpatient, there will be no more
weekly clinic visits, which over the past few weeks have become
for me uncomfortable and unproductive. My colleague whose
turn it is to manage the ward this month is now the physician
of record. He sees Noam and her parents daily, and a terrible,
unspoken collusion evolves, where we are easily able to avoid
engaging the parents in any substantial conversations. We focus
instead on the details of day-to-day management—blood counts
and electrolytes and fluids and such—and simply don't talk about
what we know will come next. All of us are complicit in avoiding
the overarching issue, the inexorable march of her disease.

Even though I'm no longer driving the day-to-day decisions,
I stop by Noam's room almost daily. But my visits are brief and
are mostly spent asking her parents minor, superficial questions
about her condition: How is Noam feeling today? How much

did she eat? After two weeks of this I begin to feel like a partici-
pant in a tragic charade that we've all, through some unspoken
accord, agreed to play out. One Thursday, I catch myself slipping out of the hospital for the weekend without even bothering to look in on Noam. Ashamed that I've gotten to the point
where I'm deliberately avoiding even the most basic interactions,
I force myself to go back up to the department. When I get to
her room, Noam is asleep in bed, her face now the color of a yel-
low highlighter—a sad sign of how far the disease has advanced
into her liver. Her mother sits by the bedside, torso twisted and
draped over the bed as she caresses one of Noam's matchstick
arms. I enter with my briefcase in hand, my not-so-subtle way of
indicating that I am just stopping by on my way out, that I have
no intention of engaging Noam's mother in another pointless
conversation. Though it's already dusk, no one has bothered to
turn the lights on in the room, and I wonder how long she has
been sitting there in the semidarkness. I put my bag down and
pull a chair over to the foot of the bed. Watching the slow rise
and fall of Noam's chest, I say nothing. Time passes, and the
room grows dimmer. I very much want to say something, but I
most certainly do not want simply to rehash the unproductive
conversations we have already had. So I just sit and watch them,
a mother cradling her limp, dying child, like some sort of modern
Pietà. After what feels like a long time, during which my mind
wanders from Michelangelo, to Rome, to plans for an upcoming
vacation abroad, Noam's mother looks up at me. I can see in the
darkening shadows where her tears have stained Noam's pillow.

"I want to ask a question," she says. She pauses before starting again. "I want to ask a question, but I am afraid I don't want
the answer. I am afraid of what you will say."

I pull my chair a bit closer, wondering if this is what we have
been waiting to hear.

"I am afraid," she says, "that there are no more treatments. I
am afraid that you will tell me that this is it."

Somehow, the right combination of mood, circumstance,

and silence has created a space that has enabled Noam's mother to open up.

We speak quietly. It's clear that we are now engaged in a very different conversation than the ones we had been having. We talk about how to make Noam feel more comfortable during this current hospital admission, and we acknowledge that we will need to think about how to make her feel comfortable down the road, as Noam's disease progresses and she gets sicker. But first she wants to have the weekend to be with Noam and to talk with her husband. We agree to sit down again on Sunday, away from Noam's bedside, to talk about and plan for what happens next.

WHEN I RETURN TO TEL AVIV at the end of each day, I hear the evening call of the muezzin, often while I'm walking or jogging by the ocean to clear my head as the waves crash along the breakers. The chaos of the day, the pressures at work, the stress of the commute, the problems of the region all seem to fade away. If I get home early enough, the lawns along the seaside promenade at the southern edge of Tel Aviv are still crowded with families from Jaffa, cooking their dinners over small coal grills. The air fills with happy chatter—Arabic, Hebrew, a smattering of English, French, and Russian. Kids are laughing and bells are jangling as a horse slowly clip-clops along, its owner hawking sunset rides. The sounds fill me with joy at being here and make me feel that, yes, I'm in the right place and doing the right thing. I sit on the roof of my apartment building as the sun goes down, watching the ocean and the lights of Jaffa in the distance, enjoying the silence and, on occasion, the sounds of life that softly fill it.

5

Home

TEL AVIV IS SOMETIMES CALLED the White City, a reference to its UNESCO (United Nations Educational, Scientific, and Cultural Organization) status as housing the largest collection of Bauhaus architecture in the world. The first apartment that I rent when I move there is in a beautiful, classic 1930s example of this style, with a big, sunny porch. But it's on the ground floor. As I'd experienced at work, Israelis are notorious for their loose approach to personal space, and when I leave open my shutters or my balcony door, it's as though anyone in the immediate vicinity has been invited into both my apartment and my life. Trying to have a serious conversation with a friend? Be prepared for the unsolicited input of your neighbor across the driveway. Spending a pleasant evening with a date? Brace yourself for feedback on your amatory techniques from that neighbor the next morning. I respond by withdrawing, keeping my shutters and porch doors closed most of the time. Before long my apartment starts to feel more like a cave than the airy open space

I had hoped for. Reluctantly, I resolve to find a place to live that affords me a bit more privacy while still managing to feel like a home.

Through a strange coincidence, the next apartment I land in is the same one that my parents had rented several years earlier while on sabbatical in Israel. They had loved the apartment, and when the rental agent they used hears that I'm looking, he tells me that the place is once again available.

I jump at the opportunity. Though relatively small, the apartment takes up the entire top floor of the building, affording me some of the privacy I crave. It has high ceilings and huge windows that look out over the city on one side, and the beach and the Mediterranean Sea on the other. It feels spacious and is filled with light. The pièce de résistance is a steep flight of internal stairs that lead up to a retractable skylight, giving me access to my own private rooftop with sweeping 360-degree views. As I settle in, I'm pleasantly surprised to come across traces of my parents' occupancy years earlier—the kitchen table, an old lamp, and even some junk mail that continues to arrive addressed to them—which gives my new apartment a familiar feel and affords me an additional sense of connection to my new home. It all seems too good to be true. Which it sort of turns out to be.

Parking is scarce in the neighborhood, so as soon as I move in I go to city hall to register for a residential parking permit. After a brief search on her computer, the clerk assisting me tells me that she can't find my apartment listed in the municipal registry.

"I'm sorry," she says, "you must be making a mistake. You must have gotten the address wrong."

Showing her my rental contract, where the address and apartment number are clearly printed, accomplishes nothing. As far as the Tel Aviv municipality is concerned, my apartment does not exist. I leave empty-handed and frustrated. A quick check of my front door when I get home confirms that I do indeed live where I think I live, so I track down the landlord to ask for his advice. After some equivocation, he confesses that my apartment was illegally added onto the building and is therefore not registered with the municipality. Like many properties in this neighborhood, which dates back to the late 1890s, the building is an inheritance that is shared among a number of relatives, and they cannot agree on how to manage it. When the landlord decided that he wanted to add a floor to the top of the building, he was unable to apply for the necessary construction permits because he didn't have the consent of all the co-owners. So he just went ahead and had it built anyway and simply ran pipes and wires for the water and electricity from the floors below. Back in New York, these kinds of shenanigans would make my landlord the lead item on the local television news and would result at best in a hefty fine and at worst (if that illegal wiring resulted in a fire that injured or killed someone) an extended stay in jail. But I'm an Israeli now, and I try not to let this kind of thing faze me. The parking permit, however, remains an issue, especially because in this neighborhood the police ticket illegally parked cars aggressively, and I can't get a permit without a properly addressed utility bill or municipal tax receipt to prove residency. My parents, who didn't have a car the year they lived here, never had to confront this issue. But I refuse to drop it, and the landlord finally grabs the rental contract from my hands, scrawls a clause across the bottom stating that all taxes and utilities are included in my monthly rent, initials it, and thrusts it back at me.

"Yih'yeh b'seder," he says, with a dismissive wave of his hand. The literal translation of this popular Hebrew phrase is "It will be okay," but it's also colloquial shorthand for "Stop worrying about it." All this succeeds in doing is making me feel more, not less, concerned. (At work I learn the Arabic equivalent, "Inshallah," or "God willing," which is delivered with a certain inflection of doubt, as if to say, "Hopefully it will be okay. But maybe not.")

Feeling like an idiot, I return to city hall with this handwritten addendum to the contract that I clearly might have just written myself. I find the same clerk on duty, and, handing her the contract, I mumble something about how the landlord says it's fine, *yih'yeh b'seder.* She glances at the contract, makes a sour face, and once again checks the computer database, as though the newly added clause may have also somehow magically altered the official registry. Unsurprisingly, she tells me again that the apartment doesn't exist. Abandoning my pride in being a dyed-in-the-wool Israeli, I revert to English, easily adopting the persona of the newly arrived innocent immigrant who doesn't comprehend what all the fuss is about. After a few minutes of her telling me the apartment doesn't exist and me insisting that the landlord says it's fine, she grows sufficiently bored or irritated.

"Fine," she says, printing out a parking sticker for me, "but next year don't forget to bring a bill." *Inshallah.*

The poorly spliced electrical wiring powering my apartment leads to frequent short circuits of my air conditioner, not a minor issue during a Tel Aviv summer. And as I undertake a more careful survey of the apartment, I notice pipes and wires with no clear purpose sticking out of the plaster here and there. Some of the walls have hairline cracks etching their way across the surface. This all serves as a frequent reminder that the apartment isn't totally aboveboard. But it does begin to feel like home, and I settle in, make it my own—and just hope that the walls don't collapse on me while I'm asleep in bed.

"Ownership" is a loaded term in this part of the world, where who was where first and who has a right to what is central to the very question of the state's existence. Some story pertaining to land and ownership seems to appear in the news every day, whether it's the rising cost of apartments in central Israel, right-wing Jews buying homes in Arab East Jerusalem, settlement expansion in the West Bank, Arabs seeking to buy homes in predominantly Jewish areas, or Arab homes that had been built in East Jerusalem without proper permits being razed by the government. The constant argument seems endless.

.   .   .

HOME COMES UP MORE than you might think in caring for
a child facing a life-threatening illness. Though a stable, functional, and loving home is important for all children, it makes
a huge difference in the experience, and possibly even the outcome, of treatment for a child with cancer. Until I moved to Israel,
I had never visited a patient at home; in America I'd never had
the opportunity to do so or felt the need to. It certainly was not a
part of my training. In Israel, I find that things are a bit different.

It's not actually a visit to a patient that first takes me to a
patient's home in Israel but, rather, a bereavement call. In accordance with religious tradition, most funerals in Israel—for Muslims and Jews alike—occur on the day of death, and I can't always
rearrange my work schedule to attend my patients' funerals. So
rather than attend some and not others (and risk insulting family members by my absence), I adopt a policy of not attending
funerals at all, but instead I try to make a condolence visit in the
days that follow. Jews sit shivah at home for seven days following
the death of an immediate family member and the Muslims' in-
home mourning period is three days, so there is usually enough
leeway to plan for a visit that won't feel rushed and during
which I can actually spend time with the family. Though many
of the families we care for are not particularly observant, almost
all adhere to at least some of the traditions of mourning, seeking comfort in the ancient, shared rituals when the rest of their
world has lost direction. Even if they don't rigorously observe
all of the mourning traditions, almost all families at least stay at
home for a number of days to receive visitors.

Dying from cancer is usually a process of slow deterioration—
of bodily function, mental integrity, and personal dignity. It also
involves the deterioration of a family's hopes and identity. Parents can no longer be their child's primary caregiver, nurturing
and protecting her in the manner that they have been doing

since before she was born. My colleagues and I—comparative strangers—now assume that role. That's one reason I have always felt that being a clinician for these children is a sacred undertaking. We not only have a window into the most private corners of the lives of our patients and their families but we also assume important roles in these lives. Grief, with its public and private elements, is very much a part of this world in which we find ourselves, both in the hospital and at home, both during the child's illness and after death. And so a family's grief becomes something in which we also share because, more often than not, they need to share it with us.

The first shivah visit I make is to the parents of Yitzchok, a little boy who died of a progressive muscle tumor while under my care. A young religious couple, they live in a modest Jerusalem neighborhood in one of the unattractive but functional buildings that were hastily thrown up by the government in the 1950s to absorb the waves of Jewish immigrants pouring into the new state from Arab countries in the Levant and North Africa. As I enter the apartment, I see Yitzchok's parents sitting in the living room on the customary low shivah stools, surrounded by a group of seated visitors. I am embarrassed when they break off their conversations to greet me. I hear murmured whispers around the room and the word *"rofei"* (doctor) is audible here and there. Rather than making me feel flattered or proud, the whispers and gestures burn like an indictment. After all, one could say we're all here because I failed in my duty as a doctor.

Someone offers me a plastic cup of juice, which I politely decline. A nurse from our department who happens to be visiting at the same time reprimands me the next day. She tells me that it's insulting for a guest not to accept at least a drink of water, which is offered as a sign of welcome. There is something appealingly biblical about this (it brings to mind Abraham, recovering from his circumcision, greeting the three angels in front of his tent), and from then on every time I am offered food or drink at a house of mourning I dutifully accept, whether I need it or not.

Yitzchok's mother and grandmother get up and insist that I accompany them to his bedroom. It has been left just as it was before his final hospital admission. They proceed to show me all of his belongings—basically toys and stuffed animals—carefully describing and telling a story about each item like shopkeepers proudly displaying their inventory. They then start flipping through a massive photo album, the sheer volume of which seems wildly at odds with Yitzchok's short life. This is a ritual I will find repeated at almost every shivah I attend. For my colleagues and me, at the end of a long and difficult day, it can at times be exhausting. Most of us want simply to express our condolences, say something kind, and then move on to the comfort of our own homes. But the truth is that we are fortunate. I would understand if we were the last people in the world that parents wanted to see while mourning their loss. But here are parents whose child has died under our care, and all they want to do is welcome us in, to show us a little bit of who their child was before he got sick. It is an act of bearing witness for them and, ultimately, for us, attesting to the fact that this was not just a patient but a person. I come to embrace this ritual, seeing my patients for one last time as their parents desperately want to remember them: as happy, beautiful children enjoying their all-too-brief lives surrounded by loving family and friends.

Most of the patients in our department who die do so in the hospital. Studies from North America suggest that given the choice, most children would choose, when possible, to die at home, with their parents and siblings at their side, surrounded by their toys and belongings and by the familiar sounds and smells of home. There is no reason to think that children here are any different. "When possible," however, is no small thing, as it means having a support system set up so that the family feels secure at home and can adequately manage the child's symptoms and any sudden problems that might arise as death approaches.

In the United States, home hospice services often fill this role, though even in the United States there are an insufficient number of hospice agencies, certainly ones with pediatric experience, to cover the needs of the entire population. Israel has an even less robust pediatric home hospice system, so our department makes do with an ad hoc system for supporting dying children and their families at home. It's not perfect, but it's better than nothing. When parents decide that they prefer to care for their child at home, our doctors and nurses try to make home visits as often as possible and try to manage the rest by phone. Our availability is limited, however, by the fact that we all have busy clinic schedules and nobody has time specifically dedicated to outpatient home care. This can generate enormous stress when a child is nearing death, as symptoms such as pain or shortness of breath may flare up without warning at any time, and a staff member may not be immediately available for a home visit or even a telephone consultation.

But we devote ourselves to this work, making every effort to provide the right kind of support when the end seems to be approaching. This often involves providing care—either by phone or in person—when we are technically off duty, at the end of a long day or on a weekend, but that's the nature of the job. Though our visits are sometimes prompted by urgent changes in the clinical picture, sometimes we check in on our sickest patients just to see how things are going, to make sure that we have a full understanding of what is happening with them. Though we can always speak with parents by phone for updates, there is no substitute for actually being in the room and evaluating the patient ourselves. Sometimes as I sit in a patient's home late in the evening, watching parents watch their dying child, with nothing in particular required of me, I wonder if I truly am accomplishing anything, if I'm truly adding anything to their care when I could just as easily be out with friends enjoying myself. But more often than not the home visits are meaningful and important, even if it takes some time for the import to become clear.

. . .

DALIA IS A FOURTEEN-YEAR-OLD GIRL who for the past two years has been receiving treatment for a slowly progressing tumor. She is now nearing the end, with no real disease-directed treatments available, and she and her family have made it clear that they wish to have her spend her final weeks at home in central Jerusalem rather than in the hospital. At the beginning we check in every few days, making sure she has enough medications for her occasional breakthrough symptoms. But as her disease progresses over the next few weeks, we intensify our management, finally placing her on a continuous intravenous infusion of medicines for pain and sedation. This is intended to provide the best comfort possible without actually hastening death; the goal is to allow Dalia to be pain-free but alert enough to continue to have meaningful interactions with her family. Like many aspects of life in Israel, the legality of how we actually do this is a bit fuzzy around the edges. I feel confident that we are providing excellent, safe medical care with the infusions. But the procedure for how the opioids are being dispensed isn't totally clear to me. At Hadassah, as in American hospitals, opioid medications (morphine and its derivatives) are supposed to be carefully regulated so as to prevent misuse, such as illegal sale or abuse by a staff member. Despite that, I've noticed a large stash of vials rolling around in the trunk of the car of a colleague who is caring for Dalia that in the United States would likely be enough to get her arrested for intent to sell. I'm not sure how she managed to have it dispensed by the pharmacy and, worse still, she doesn't seem to be keeping a record of how much has been used. It's also unclear whether we are covered by malpractice insurance outside the hospital and what formal guidelines we are following, especially since a large part of our care is providing guidance to Dalia's parents, who then adjust the medications themselves. In the hospital we carefully adjust the rate of infusion via computerized pump, so that we know exactly how much medication each patient is getting. In Dalia's case, we don't have a pump set up at her home, so we simply inject the medications into a bag of IV fluids that is running into her port and change the rate of infusion by adjusting a plastic clamp on the tubing. Without a precise knowledge of how much medication we are administering, we modify the drip based on her clinical appearance. The one time I ask about malpractice insurance I am told not to worry: *yih'ye b'seder.* I understand that the most important thing here is taking care of Dalia's symptoms, so I go along with it.

After several weeks of this I'm in the clinic one day when Dalia's mother calls in a panic, telling me to come quickly. "She's going," she says through her tears. A nurse and I jump into her car to make the short drive together. We arrive to find Dalia unconscious, with the irregular breathing that clearly signals impending death. We are there during the last hour of Dalia's life, slipping in and out of her room to make sure she is comfortable while her parents remain at her side. After she has passed away, as we gather in the living room to fill out the death certificate and notify the burial society, there is a moment where I find myself alone in the kitchen with Dalia's mother. This is an Orthodox family, and in the more than two years that I have cared for her daughter I have never had any form of physical contact whatsoever with this woman. (Her husband, on the other hand, goes out of his way to shake my hand hello and goodbye at each encounter; it's almost as if he feels he's doing this on behalf of his entire family.) But now, in her raw grief at her child's death, she throws her arms around me, hugging me tightly and whispering her thanks. I'm surprised but pleased by her kindness and the gesture of acceptance. After all we have been through together, I feel that this family regards me as one of their own.

Over the next hour Dalia's siblings, summoned from school, filter in. They go into the bedroom to say goodbye to their sister, emerging to comfort their parents and each other. Dalia's death was not unexpected, but there is always a shock of finality, even for me, when it does happen. No matter how prepared a family is, there is a recognition that the particular dynamic that is unique to this family has been changed forever; one stage of their existence has ended and another is about to begin. A hole has been cut into Dalia's family, and though it may never truly be filled, as I watch her parents and siblings interact I can already see the scar tissue beginning to form over it, the still-bleeding wound being stanched by their love for one another. I find myself thinking about my own family, and missing them. My sister, who made aliyah several years before I did, lives in the north of Israel, too far away for me just to drop in whenever I want to, and my parents and brother are still in the United States. The day has been draining, and I am looking forward to getting back to Tel Aviv. But this scene, and the embrace by Dalia's mother in the kitchen, make me all the more aware that I will be going back to an empty home.

I'm in my mid-thirties, and I know that time is passing. This marks the first period in my life when it's occurred to me that, despite all of the opportunities that still lie ahead, some doors may be closing for me. Each time I hear about the wedding of an ex-girlfriend or about an old friend who has settled down and started having kids, I realize how far away I am from creating my own family. Even though I'm not entirely sure that this is what I want at this point in my life, when I see families like Dalia's I can't deny the twinge of jealousy that stabs me. I quietly watch from a corner as Dalia's parents and siblings embrace one another, and I long for that same love, that same intimacy. There's something slightly voyeuristic about the way I watch this family deal with their sorrow, a comfort that I take in watching them comfort one another. For a brief moment I try to convince myself that I am part of this family's experience. Their commitment and resolve stand in stark contrast to my own bachelor's life, to what I'm left with when I flee from one relationship to another at the slightest hint of a challenge. It awakens all sorts of complex feelings inside me.

And yet there is also comfort in my solitude. In having my own space. In doing things my own way, right or wrong. After a day like this, when I return home exhausted and spent, I am in many ways grateful not to have to consider, engage with, or just be there for someone else. And then there are the nights when I wake in the dark, listening to the wind and painfully aware that something is missing in my life. I am eager for the morning, when I will again experience life through the joy and sorrow of others, through the simulacrum of a family that my work life has become.

FOR SOME PATIENTS, home may not always feel like the safest or most comfortable place to be. When faced with advancing illness, some children and their parents in fact prefer the hospital, where they can be supported and comforted by the staff around the clock. Providing options is important. At this critical time in the life of a family, when so many options are being taken away, preserving choices for how and where a patient's final days are spent is almost an act of defiance: death may be inevitable, but the family will, as much as possible, maintain control over what happens between now and then, including where it happens.

Unfortunately, the option to remain comfortably at home is not one that we are able to offer many of our Palestinian patients. While our staff at Hadassah can to some degree provide at-home care for our Israeli patients, as Israeli citizens we are not legally permitted to enter Palestinian towns and villages in Area A and Area B in the West Bank (as defined by the 1995 Oslo II Accords) to provide the same care for our Palestinian patients. As a dual Israeli and American citizen, I always have the option of flashing my American passport if need be, but when I ask col-

leagues, they tell me it's a risky proposition and that neither the
Israelis nor the Palestinians would be willing to guarantee my
safety. Conversely, friends and extended family of our Palestinian patients in those areas can't enter Israel without a special
permit. So the parents of dying Palestinian children under our
care are forced to make a terrible choice. They may remain in
the hospital, with the full support of our staff, with all the necessary medications and equipment but without the company of
family and friends, or they may bring their child home to die,
surrounded by friends and family but without our team present to provide the symptom relief and pain management that
would be available at Hadassah. It's a choice no parent should
ever have to make, and it's hard for me to understand why some
accommodation, some exception to the rules, cannot be made
by the Israeli government and the Palestinian Authority for a
child who's dying of cancer. I can stand on a ridge just above the
hospital and look out at nearby Palestinian towns in Area A and
Area B. They are close enough so that when conflict flares we
can easily strike each other with artillery and rifle fire, but I cannot cross that short distance to provide comfort for a dying child.

Arabs who live in East Jerusalem are not subject to the same
travel restrictions as those living in the West Bank. This eastern
half of the city was seized by Jordan during the War of Independence in 1948, but after the Six-Day War it came under Israel's
control, along with the rest of the West Bank. In 1980 the Israeli
government formally annexed East Jerusalem to the western part
of the city. This area is populated almost entirely by Arabs (there
are a bit more than a half-dozen Jewish neighborhoods here and
there, including Mount Scopus), but how exactly to classify the
Arabs of East Jerusalem—and how they classify themselves—is a
complex issue. The answer you get depends on who and where
you're asking. Though East Jerusalem now falls under Israeli civil
jurisdiction and the inhabitants are eligible for Israeli citizenship,
most of the Arabs who live in this area do not register as such,

even though they are subject to Israeli law and dependent on Israeli civil services such as water management and trash collection. And regardless of their feelings about being Israeli citizens, our patients who live in East Jerusalem have their healthcare covered by the Israeli national health insurers, just like any other Israeli.

In one of these East Jerusalem neighborhoods, in the valley below the walled Old City of Jerusalem, lives Yassin, a sixteen-year-old with a rare tumor in his chest that recurs shortly after his initial chemotherapy treatment. I am introduced to him and his parents after the tumor has shown no response to further therapy and it's clear that progression is inevitable. There are no more interventions to offer, and we are meeting to discuss how to manage what time remains for him. His parents have brought along his newborn sister. I am both reassured and taken aback by her presence, by this new life cooing away in the midst of a room thick with the talk of death. She is, on the one hand, a comforting if clichéd reminder that life does renew itself. On the other hand, as I look at her I can't help but imagine newborn Yassin being cradled by this same woman sixteen years ago, as his parents happily planned his future, never imagining they would end up in a place like this. I wonder if his mother is thinking the same thing. She holds the baby tight, as though both drawing comfort from her and shielding her from us and from the world we represent.

Yassin declares pretty quickly that he wants to spend as little time in the hospital as possible. He's always been friendly and appreciative of our efforts, despite our failure to cure his cancer. But he's clearly not interested in spending any more of his time here than is absolutely necessary. We decide that he should come in just for weekly checkups, but as his disease progresses we agree that these visits make less and less sense. Because Yassin lives in East Jerusalem we can make home visits, and we resolve to do our best to provide care for him there.

I've seen Yassin's neighborhood many times before, but only from a distance. There is a beautiful promenade along the terraced ridges of West Jerusalem that has been crafted from rose-gold Jerusalem stone and is bordered with cypress trees, rosemary bushes, and lush flower beds. You can look down into the valley and see the walls of the Old City and the golden dome of the Al-Aqsa Mosque that rises above it, and farther east, the green slopes of Mount Scopus and the Mount of Olives. You can also look down onto a jumble of tightly packed neighborhoods that spill down from the easternmost side of the Old City and fill the Kidron Valley. Here and there a large Israeli flag marks a home that has been bought by right-wing Jews in their slow but steady attempt to change the character of these Arab neighborhoods. They are a reminder that this is an area where violence could explode at any moment. I know the names of these neighborhoods from my patients' charts and from hearing them mentioned on television news programs—Silwan, Ras el-Amud, Jabel Mukaber—and I try to pronounce them with the proper Arabic intonations, now that I'm a local boy. But there is no denying that in my mouth the names still feel foreign, even forbidden, no matter how many flags we plant in their soil.

The Kidron Valley got its name from the stream mentioned in the Bible that runs through it. Some say that it's the area that the biblical book of Joel refers to as Emek Yehoshafat ("the Valley Where God Judges"), where during the Messianic era there will be a settling of accounts with the nations that oppressed the Jews during the millennia of exile from the Land. In any case, I'm about to see it up close for the first time, as I prepare for my first home visit to Yassin.

I go with a nurse who has been there before and who offers to drive so that I don't get lost in the narrow alleyways and unmarked lanes. As we reach the crest of the ridge that marks the end of the Jewish neighborhoods, we start a steep descent down narrow switchbacks into the valley. Near the start of the descent we pass a heavily fortified post manned by border police. The government may say that we are all residents of one united Jerusalem, but it's obvious that some neighborhoods get treated differently than others. As we continue driving, it is as though we are going back hundreds of years in time. The road is broken and full of potholes, and once we reach the floor of the valley it becomes impossibly dusty and narrow, the homes and shops closing in tightly on either side. There is barely enough space for cars to squeeze by. Flowing around our slow-moving vehicle are a mix of pedestrians, goats, donkeys, and chickens. Shops open directly onto the road, close enough so that I could reach out the car window and touch their wares. Merchants have their goods laid out in the sun and dust, displaying crates of fruits and vegetables, or suspending chains from which hunks of unidentifiable meat hang, impaled on large, mean-looking hooks. Looking back up toward the ridge, I see a river of garbage spilling down the barren slope, as though a reservoir of refuse has burst its dam. Anyone who claims that Jerusalem is undivided has never been down here.

After several twists and turns we start up the opposite side of the valley and soon arrive at Yassin's home. The whole trip has taken less than ten minutes. We are within hiking distance of the cafés and shops of upscale West Jerusalem neighborhoods such as the German Colony and Baka, but in every other respect we are a world away.

The apartment building is an unadorned, rectangular three-story building of poured concrete, and iron bars protruding from the top indicate that it's still a work in progress. The buildings in the neighborhood are largely indistinguishable from one another, most looking like they are either still under construction or in the process of falling apart. Like most homes here, Yassin's has a large black plastic water tank sitting on the roof. The nurse tells me that the water supply from the Jerusalem municipality is undependable and is often shut off without warning. The tanks provide a reserve supply, just in case. The area in front of the building is a dirt lot, and as we park there I note that the ground floor of the building has been converted to a small stable. A horse pokes its long snout in our direction out a half-open door.

We get out of the car and I look around and up toward the valley's eastern ridge. It doesn't look all that different than the opposite side from which we've just come, except for one thing—a gray concrete wall that runs along the ridge, rising up starkly against the bright blue sky. It's a segment of the separation barrier, the wall around the West Bank that the government began to build in response to terrorist incursions into Israeli cities during the Second Intifada. Yassin lives, quite literally, in the shadow of the wall. Had his village been situated just a few miles to the east, on the other side of that wall, we might not have been able to make this sort of home visit.

Yassin's parents welcome us in. The house is sparsely furnished but neat, with thin, colorful area rugs scattered throughout providing some contrast to the concrete floors. Sunlight pours into the living room, but I notice that only a few of the windows actually contain panes of glass; the rest are simply open spaces with rough, unfinished edges that have been cut into the walls. Yassin's father appears embarrassed when he sees me scanning the place, and he quickly apologizes and tells me that the apartment is still being worked on. He gives me a tour, pointing out where he will be adding walls, cabinets, and decorative items. We end the tour in Yassin's bedroom, which, in contrast to the rest of the house, appears to be completely finished, well-furnished, and sweetly decorated. It feels like we have stepped into a totally different home. Yassin is lying in bed, propped up with several pillows, a sure sign that his lungs are by now so filled with tumor and fluid that lying flat is impossible. Next to his bed an IV pump on a pole quietly hums away. The bedside table is neatly stacked with boxes and bottles of pills. We arrange several chairs and sit and chat for a while, making sure that Yassin is comfortable, that he has enough of a supply of medications, that the IV pump delivering pain medication (in this case we've managed to get an actual digital pump) is working properly. We make small talk and drink fresh carob juice, which his mother insists is imbued with powerful restorative properties. Through the window I can see clear across the valley to that promenade in West Jerusalem where I have so often walked and jogged and wondered about the villages down here and the people who live in them.

Yassin lives for weeks beyond our expectations. As some studies now suggest, once aggressive disease-directed therapy has been stopped and more attention is paid to comfort and quality of life, some end-stage patients may live not just more comfortably but also longer than expected. I am convinced that part of what has kept Yassin alive has to do with his not coming to our clinic, where we would have tinkered with his body in ways that we couldn't at his home—drawing blood, giving fluids, correcting electrolytes, trying to fix the unfixable. Instead of addressing lab values and blood tests, we help support Yassin's comfort in his bedroom, adjusting medications based only on his reports of symptoms such as pain and nausea.

The night that Yassin passes away I am abroad at a medical conference. The nurse, called to his home to help manage the symptoms of active dying and to support the family, is stopped by the border police at the security checkpoint.

"Are you crazy?" a policeman asks her when she tells him where she's headed. "It's not safe down there at night."

They insist on sending a jeep full of policemen to accompany her into the valley. United Jerusalem, I think again wryly when the nurse tells me the story upon my return. I feel that we have accomplished something by enabling Yassin to die at home. But I wonder what you call a home with an irregular water supply, with windows that look out onto a flowing river of trash, with a bunch of guys with guns sitting in your living room to protect the nurse who has come to minister to your dying child. When you live in the shadow of a concrete separation barrier.

When I return to my apartment that evening, I survey my belongings, my ever-growing library that I insist on dragging with me each time I move, the trinkets collected on various vacations, and I wonder if all of it makes this place *my* home. I love the city I live in, the city I work in, the land around me, but now that I'm actually living here, I am all too often aware of its heartbreaking complexities, its intractable problems, and I wonder if it will ever truly feel like home.

6

The Proximity of Danger

MOST CHILDREN WITH CANCER SURVIVE. There are, of course, some diagnoses that carry with them almost no chance for cure (a colleague of mine once asserted that when oncologists say that odds are "less than 20 percent," it's only because they're unable to bring themselves to say "zero"). But for the most part, children who have been diagnosed with cancer do very well under treatment, and their cancers do not recur—a fact that we try to emphasize when talking with families of newly diagnosed patients.

Despite the good outcomes, however, most of our treatments are still fairly inelegant and imprecise, and carry with them not just the risks of short-term side effects but also of long-term damage. The problem lies with the fact that most chemotherapies are very blunt weapons, killing *any* rapidly dividing cells in the body, the foremost example of which is cancer cells.

Unfortunately, there are many other rapidly dividing cells in our bodies that should be dividing in order to do their jobs.

But this also makes them targets of chemotherapy—innocent bystanders killed in the cross fire. These include cells at the roots of hair (their death results in baldness), in the lining of the mouth (their death results in oral ulcers), and in the bone marrow (their death results in low blood counts and a compromised immune system). There are also long-term risks, such as organ damage. And in a particularly tragic piece of irony, many chemotherapy treatments can also cause a type of cell damage that, down the road, spurs other cells in the body to become cancerous. These secondary cancers are usually much harder to treat than the original cancer, and are often lethal. Most chemotherapy also carries with it the possibility of impaired fertility in the future; in fact, some of our treatments are so intensive that we know from the outset that the patient being treated will almost certainly be rendered infertile.

Hearing about a potential loss of fertility shortly after learning of a cancer diagnosis can be, for our young patients and their parents, a second devastating blow. This is especially true among observant Jews and Muslims, for whom having children is such an important part of the culture and where alternatives such as adoption and sperm or egg donation may not be widely accepted. In order to mitigate, as much as possible, the risk of infertility, we generally offer sperm banking for boys who have reached puberty and ovarian cryopreservation (the removal and freezing of part or all of an ovary) for even very young girls. We frame these options in optimistic terms, as a way of looking at the glass as half full. Yes, our treatments are likely to cause long-lasting damage, but we are hopeful that with the help of these treatments our patients will be alive for many years to come and will someday want children of their own.

With time I become more adept at these conversations, but the very first time I walk into a room to discuss sperm banking with a new patient, I realize too late that I completely lack the necessary vocabulary in Hebrew. The patient is Hayim, a fifteen-year-old Modern Orthodox Jewish boy. He is a patient of one of my female colleagues, and though I've never met him before, she feels that he might be more comfortable having this discussion with another male. His parents, still reeling from the news themselves, have given me permission to talk with him alone.

Hayim sits across the desk from me in the exam room, adjusting the large knitted *kippah* that covers most of his head. His face is pale underneath his scattered acne, and though he gives me a smile, I can tell he's scared. He learned about the cancer diagnosis only yesterday, and now he's alone in a room with this new doctor who's about to give him who-knows-what additional news. He's just approaching the age where he should be thinking about plans for his army service, not about hair loss and infertility.

I make it through the introduction to the topic reasonably well, explaining in simple Hebrew terms how chemotherapy can affect fertility. I also tell him, trying to sound hopeful, that I think he will do well with the treatment and that I want him to be able to have children in the future. The way we can ensure that, I explain, is to take some of his sperm and store it in a freezer until he is married and ready to have children.

"Okay," he says, nodding. It doesn't seem to me that he has figured out where I'm going with this.

Long pause.

"So," I continue, "we would need you to produce some sperm for us in a cup. Alone, of course," I quickly add.

Hayim looks at me blankly. Either he has no idea what I'm talking about, what I'm asking him to do, or I'm being too indirect and need to explain things a bit more precisely. The only problem is that I have no idea what the Hebrew word for masturbation is, and no clue about how to explain it to an Orthodox boy, for whom masturbation is absolutely forbidden—with certain exceptions, such as this one. I feel like I'm trapped in a perverse, X-rated word game as I try to explain the act without actually naming it. At one point, at a complete loss for words, I find myself starting to make a commonly used hand gesture, but I quickly stop, embarrassed by the fact that the gesture has crude sexual connotations that seem inappropriate for a clinical discussion with a new patient. But somewhere along the line I appear to have made myself understood to Hayim. Something clicks and he rescues me by suddenly nodding vigorously and saying, repeatedly, "No problem, no problem." I excuse myself to go make the necessary arrangements but first scurry off to ask Mickey for pointers on vocabulary.

DESPITE OUR FOCUS ON HOPE, some of our patients do, unfortunately, get to the point where there is no more room for us to waffle about a prognosis, where we have to address the fact that there is truly no longer a realistic expectation for a cure. I often wonder when, over the course of a series of failed treatments, it begins to occur to a patient and his family that he might not survive his illness. Doctors can actually be an obstacle in this process. Yes, hope is important. But conveying a realistic outlook is also critical in helping patients and families make choices about treatment options and think about the future. All families come into our department understanding that it is possible that their child will die of his disease; after all, the sign at the door announces that it's the Department of Oncology. But as the chance of cure grows more remote, how do patients and their families arrive at the point of truly understanding that there will be no cure, that this disease will ultimately and unavoidably end the patient's life? I can tell you how a lot of doctors get there: gradually, reluctantly, careening back and forth between optimism and despair, watching the worsening numbers with sinking hearts, observing the clinical signs in our patients that tell us that our highest hopes and best-laid plans are faltering. And then we redouble our efforts to find alternative treatments. We do not want to accept our patients' mortality any more than they do. I have seen colleagues examine CT scans and MRIs of new patients, trace on a screen the luminous outline of brain tumors so definitive and lethal that no confirmatory biopsy is even necessary, and then, astonishingly, begin to discuss treatment options with the patient and her family.

Occasionally there are defeats that strike suddenly, like a biological Pearl Harbor, when children who were making progress with their treatments are suddenly overcome by bleeding, infections, or shock. In these instances your fear arrives in a flash, a cold spear thrust into your belly, a numbness that buckles your legs. This is it, you say to yourself. Despite everything you've done, your patient is going to die. But far more often the loss of hope, the acknowledgment of defeat, is a gradual process that sneaks up on you. And once it's there, you're left trying to manage that awful gap in time between when you know you are going to lose a patient and the patient's actual death.

I watch my patients and their parents closely, trying to understand what they do during that period. Regardless of how certain we are of a patient's inevitable death, it seems like most parents never completely lose hope that their child will, somehow, be cured of her disease. Even as they assure us that they know what is coming, many parents and patients continue to ask about new or alternative treatments—for example, phase-one trials.

WE SPEND A GREAT DEAL OF TIME in medicine, especially in subspecialties that deal with life-threatening illness, worrying about how to soften the blow of bad news, trying not to "destroy hope." This is often just an avoidance technique on our part. It delays a difficult conversation that could and should have occurred much earlier and leaves patients and their families unprepared for events that will unfold whether we want to acknowledge them or not. The earlier we begin to engage families in discussions about illnesses that are potentially life-threatening or about end-of-life management, the more time they have to think about options and make decisions that are appropriate for their situations. I've never had a family complain that I brought up difficult decision making too early, but I've heard plenty of families lament that they waited until it was too late to plan for what might be in the best interests of a dying patient.

Clinicians are also human, and fallible. I have caught myself, in the midst of difficult conversations with parents about their child who is without a doubt going to die, adding the qualifying phrase "almost certainly"—a vain and sometimes counterproductive attempt to leave myself and my patient just a tiny bit of room for that miracle that we know won't happen.

But in whatever terms we choose to cushion it, however long we delay in actually saying it, what never ceases to amaze me is the strength, dignity, and grace that most patients display when we tell them that they are going to die.

I MEET CHAVA, AN ULTRA-ORTHODOX WOMAN in her early twenties who has just been diagnosed with a rare sarcoma, not long after her wedding. Though it appears to have originated in her chest wall, it has already spread throughout both lungs. She arrives for our first meeting together with her new husband. She is pale, and her wig is slightly askew—probably because she is so newly married she has not yet had all that much practice in placing it on her head. She radiates an air of fortitude and positivity. Her husband, an affable young yeshiva student, looks far more scared.

As I take her history, I begin to suspect that Chava has been aware for some time that something was wrong. The lump on her back, her shortness of breath, the pains that would wake her at night—she couldn't have missed it all. But she remained focused on her wedding, determined not to let anything get in the way of the most important day of her life. As it turns out, because Chava's tumor is a particularly aggressive one, had she sought medical care prior to the wedding, it would not likely have changed the outcome. And she wouldn't have had a husband to help her through her yearlong treatment.

Over the course of that year we beat back each recurrence by changing the chemotherapy regimen, hoping each time for a more permanent response and, eventually, for that miracle. But the day finally arrives when we run out of new therapies, and I have no clever answers to Chava's determined "Okay, what treatment comes next?" I am sitting in my clinic office with Chava and her husband on the evening that the scan results come back, the three of us talking quietly over her deep, wet coughs. They were aware, of course, after each recurrence that the odds for a complete recovery were getting worse and that with each recurrence we were left with fewer and fewer treatment options. But now, with this evidence of the latest treatment failure and with nothing left to offer but some mild oral chemotherapy in the hope that it will slow progression, I begin to discuss with them the end. Not so much the details—the nitty-gritty of where Chava would die, how it would look, what we could do to palliate symptoms—all that could wait. Rather, this is the moment when our conversation formally turns from what we can do to stave off death to acknowledging its inevitability and our need to begin discussing how we will plan for it.

They sit across from me, both of them ashen-faced. From our first meeting Chava's face has always had a gray pallor, but now her husband's color matches hers. When they leave with plans to return in two days for follow-up, I think there is a reasonable chance that I will never see them again, despite the relationship that we have developed. Having exhausted all hope that medicine has to offer, they might now turn to their rabbis, seeking the kind of let-the-facts-be-damned hope that religious belief offers.

I also worry that, despite the ultra-Orthodox disavowal of the Internet, they or someone close to them will take to scouring the Web for solutions. The Internet has been a boon to those who would take advantage of the vulnerable, who would prey on the weak and the desperate, taking money in exchange for modern-day snake oil remedies.

But on the appointed day Chava and her husband return. I greet them in my office, ready to be faced with questions about treatments that they have dug up in their desperation. Or for them to act as though our last conversation hadn't happened, or at least try to minimize it and pretend it wasn't all that bad. I am wrong. They hold hands and smile at me through their tears. They don't ask for miracles or for more tests; they just want to know what we do now.

The degree of resolve that people can muster even in the worst circumstances is incredibly humbling to witness. How do my patients—and their families—continue to function when they know, incontrovertibly, that within a matter of weeks or months they are going to die? The simple response, the one I hear most often, is *Well, what's the alternative?* I understand what they mean by that, but the truth is that there are alternatives, and we do occasionally see them. There are parents who fight openly with each other in my office when I'm trying to discuss end-of-life care; parents who are in such deep despair that they just stare at me, incapable of responding; and parents who simply stop showing up for appointments, refusing to discuss what comes next. But most seem to be able to tap into some secret reserve of strength, one that I'm not sure I myself have. Some patients and their families even seem to gain strength during this period, supporting one another with a quiet courage and dignity. Philosophers and theologians have expended much ink arguing that the process of moving from despair to acceptance can be transformative, that an individual may in fact emerge with a greater and stronger sense of self. But how this happens, how people not only avoid falling into despair but actually grow stronger eludes me. I watch each family intently, trying to divine just what it is that makes people so resilient.

THE CLOSEST I'VE EVER COME to facing my own mortality was probably on a trip very far from Israel, while high-altitude trekking in India. Early in my medical training, on a whim, I had gone on a two-week climb in the mountains of Nepal. There didn't seem to be anything particularly dangerous about the trip, though in retrospect I suppose accidents can happen anywhere. But the risk of such accidents feels distant when one is climbing on a well-trodden path, and such fears are easily pushed aside. What I did discover on that trip, though, was an addiction to the adrenaline rush that comes with trekking at high altitude.

Many have written about the sublime nature of mountain ranges, the awe and terror they evoke. Edmund Burke, in his treatise on the sublime, suggests that part of our attraction to the sublime is the proximity of fear and danger. As I pushed myself higher and higher with each successive trip, I became more aware of the potential dangers, some perhaps proximal and exaggerated in my mind and some very real.

Setting out on each ascent, as the effects of the altitude kicked in—splitting headaches, loss of appetite, sleepless nights in flimsy tents, hips aching against the frozen ground—I would curse myself and wonder why I was wasting a vacation on this sort of unpleasantness when there were so many beaches in the world where I could be relaxing instead. But each trip was also transcendent: the sweep of snowcapped mountains, the wonder of stumbling onto a tiny village in the middle of nowhere, the beauty of narrow strips of elegantly manicured gardens perched on a distant mountain, graceful marks of humanity tucked into the vastness of nature. Words cannot capture the mystical, ecstatic, exhausted moment, the undeniable sacredness of coming to the top of a windswept pass after a hard ascent and finding a small makeshift shrine, a simple pile of rocks with colored prayer flags flapping, placed there to honor the local deity. I returned from each trip depleted in body but at the same time aching to go farther, to places higher and more remote.

By the end of my second year at Hadassah I was bent on breaking 19,700 feet (6,000 meters). One of the problems with planning this sort of a vacation is that the higher you climb, the more time you need to factor in for acclimatization. Ladakh, a region of India that juts up onto the Himalayan plateau amid China, Pakistan, and Tibet, was one of the few places where I thought I could do this in less than two weeks. I began my acclimatization with a few days of strolling through Leh, the largest town in the area, drinking tea on the roof of the local guesthouse and nursing a mild altitude headache while taking in the stunning views of the nearby mountains, including the peak I would be climbing.

I had hoped to take my time on the climb, allowing for better acclimatization by not ascending too much on any given day. But because I needed support staff, a guide, and horses, it seemed wiser to sign on with a small group of European climbers who were already organizing a trip, even though they would be climbing faster than I had planned.

The trek was magnificent. In scenery straight out of the movies, we hiked across trackless valleys dwarfed by looming walls of snowcapped mountains. We leapfrogged over icy rivulets of snowmelt that ran across the moss-and-rock-carpeted ground. An impossibly blue sky spread out above it all, stray clouds casting huge shadows across the landscape. Hypnotized by the rhythm of my footsteps, I sank into my own thoughts. It was so much easier to contemplate thorny subjects like work, relationships, and the general frustrations of life while on this mountain, where they were just theoretical abstractions.

We reached base camp, the final stop before the push to

the summit, at midday on the third day in, and I knew I was in trouble. I already had a splitting headache from the altitude, and though we had a few hours to rest, there was still a lot of altitude left to gain that night. During the afternoon the sky had changed from turquoise to an ominous steel gray. Light snow flurries, beautiful and threatening, drifted down, and the air had turned piercingly cold. I spent the afternoon in my tent, forcing down water and ibuprofen against my growing nausea, hoping I would feel better after midnight, when we were due to set out for the summit. I knew that the degree to which I was feeling ill was already a sign that I should probably move to lower ground, but not thinking clearly (itself a sign of altitude sickness), I convinced myself that a quick ascent and return wouldn't add any substantial risk.

Just after midnight the guide roused us from our tents for porridge and tea. The group lined up outside, and by the light of our headlamps we checked each other's gear, making sure poles, crampons, and ice axes were all well secured to our packs. The sky above was black and starless, and the only sign that anything existed in the world beyond the halo of our lamps was a small row of lights bobbing high above us, a group of trekkers who had gotten a head start and were now traversing a path higher up the mountain. I took one last dose of painkiller and filed out with the group. The cold night was silent except for the sound of our heavy breathing and our boots crunching on snow and ice.

In my memory, the hours that followed are a long, dark blur interspersed with brief moments of clarity. I recall wading through snowdrifts in a dark so impenetrable that there were moments when I thought I was the only person alive in the world; watching the guide strap crampons onto my boots before we began a steep ascent up a wall of iced-over snow and rock; and occasionally stopping to force down a mouthful of energy gel and water despite my utter lack of appetite. Faces passed in and out of my headlamp's glow, and our small group became more and more scattered in the dark, each person becoming increasingly absorbed in his or her own efforts. At one point I heard a disembodied voice, high above, cry out for his mother.

As dawn approached I was able to see the ridgeline above, and I watched the sky slowly brighten as I dragged myself up the final few feet. From there the path continued upward, less steeply but now cutting along the razor back of the mountain via a narrow path paved with sharp rocks and ice, and bracketed by a precipitous drop on either side. I stumbled along, slipping here and there, trying to take in the scene around me as the sunrise broke over the mountains, while still maintaining enough focus on each step to keep from tumbling over the side.

Just shy of the summit I stopped. All of my senses were dulled and my brain felt fuzzy. My head was pounding with an altitude headache. I looked around, gazing down at the drop, not understanding how I had actually managed to haul myself up those slopes. Every muscle in my body felt depleted, every breath hurt, and I wasn't sure which end of my gastrointestinal tract was going to give up first. It suddenly occurred to the small part of my brain that was still functioning properly that I might not be able to make it back down, that this time I might have gone too far. We were already well above the clouds, a thick, billowy mass flowing out to the horizon, pierced here and there by icy peaks. The whole world seemed to be nothing but snowy crags floating on a sea of clouds. It was sublime. I turned around to try to make it back down.

The group I had gone up with was completely scattered by this time, so I started down on my own. The sun was now fully up, but the return to camp remains even more of a blur in my memory than the ascent—a big white snowy blur instead of an inky-black dark blur. Rather than retrace my steps all the way back down, I chose the fastest way down that I could see. Ignoring the path along the ridgeline I had just come up, I dropped onto my bottom and slid straight down the wall of ice and rock, slowing and controlling my descent as much as possible with my ice ax. I must have slid down in minutes what had taken me hours to climb up. Had I not felt so sick and scared, it might have been fun.

The glissade down brought me to the edge of a huge snow-field branching off into several valleys that appeared identical. Because we had come up at night, there were no recognizable landmarks to guide me back, nothing to point me with certainty in the right direction. The sun was high in the sky, and the clouds and mist had mostly burned off. The surface of the snowpack was melting, and there were no tracks to follow. In the bright sunlight the entire landscape appeared to be on fire, sparkling with melting snow and ice. I chose a direction simply to keep moving, and, slogging across the field, I realized that if I was heading down into the wrong valley I might well die.

I don't know how close I came to not making it. I did manage to choose the correct route down, but there was at least one point during my descent when, sick and exhausted, I very seriously thought about just lying down in the snow and going to sleep. When I finally stumbled back into camp I dropped to my hands and knees and retched up all of the water and energy gel I had been trying to force down all night. I spent the rest of the day and that night mostly dozing in my tent, waking every now and then to try to drink something so as to get some sugar into my body, only to vomit after a few minutes now that more advanced altitude sickness had kicked in. After I threw up three juice boxes, the guide refused to give me any more, saying it was a waste of perfectly good juice. Instead he brought me boiled water that had come from a nearby stream, with bits of grass and dirt still swirling in it.

To most people this might all just sound like terrible, self-inflicted punishment. But it was also beautiful and challenging, cleansing and reaffirming. Peter Matthiessen described it perfectly in *The Snow Leopard,* his book about his Himalayan trek: "Perhaps this dread of transience explains our greed for the few gobbets of raw experience in modern life, why violence is libidinous, why lust devours us, why soldiers choose not to forget their days of horror: we cling to such extreme moments, in which we seem to die, yet are reborn.... My foot slips on a narrow ledge: in that split second, as needles of fear pierce heart and temples, eternity intersects with present time. Thought and action are not different, and stone, air, ice, sun, fear, and self are one."

I used to think I went on these trips to get away from everything I saw at work. But now I wonder if in some ways I'm not also seeking to try to better understand how my patients face their own fears and how they cope with the knowledge that they will soon die. It is, of course, a very different sort of confrontation. In my situation, what I am reacting to is completely self-imposed, and the threat of danger is very different from what my patients face. But I find that there is something about the nature of the extreme altitude, about the mountains themselves, and about the danger and the beauty of my encounters with them that brings me closer to God and to my own feelings of mortality.

I am drawn to the mountains for some of the same reasons I am drawn to oncology, for some of the same reasons I am drawn to the most difficult—and some would say the saddest—of our cases at Hadassah. In all of these realms I am still seeking answers to the questions that started me on this journey. Here in the mountains, or at a dying child's bedside, or sitting across from a young couple holding each other's hands and facing the loss of their world together, I learn to experience wonder—an acknowledgment, almost mystical in nature, that even if I will never be able to figure out why terrible things happen to good and innocent people, I do understand that there is some force, whether it's an omnipotent divine being or the irrepressible human spirit, that gives life meaning. Being allowed into the lives of others at such fragile moments is a gift. And despite the sometimes harrowing things I see, my faith may wobble but it doesn't ever fail completely. The souls of my patients seem to be like gemstones—fracture them and all you really do is produce another, more complex structure that reflects and refracts the experience of life, of the divine, more beautifully. When Moses asks God to reveal Himself on the mountain, God tells him that he cannot see His face and live, but that if Moses hides himself in the cleft of a rock God will pass by and Moses will see His back, the reflection of His glory as He passes by. Here on my mountain, with the sun breaking through the clouds and sparkling endlessly across the sea of icy peaks, or in the hospital watching families staggering under the relentless blows of life yet somehow managing to hold it together, or simply living in a land where so many different communities seek meaning in the face of tragedy and despair, I see the reflection of God passing by and I feel wonder.

WHEN MY PATIENTS ASK ME about strength and hope, as they often do, I still don't feel I have a great answer. In fact, I look to them for answers. Many of my colleagues talk about the idea of reframing hope. In other words, when hope for a cure is lost one can redefine what one is hoping for. But this always feels hollow to me, like patting someone on the back for winning a second-place prize. Not that those other goals are not valuable, but is there really a runner-up prize if first place is a cure?

I seek my own answers, perhaps foolishly, in high icy passes, in trying to arrive at some sense of what it feels like to be off the map with no clear plan. I want to ask my patients and their families what gives them strength. But something holds me back. I'm not sure if it's embarrassment, or a concern that it will sound like prying, or a fear that, in asking, I will force an acknowledgment that they are more lost to despair than I want to believe. Maybe if I knew where they found this strength I could help to buttress it, shore up their defenses. Maybe I would be able to tap into those resources for myself.

7

The Forces That Give Us Meaning

My PERSONAL STRUGGLE WITH THEODICY obviously did not resolve itself upon my arrival in Israel. The heavens did not part, and there was no ray of divine light shining down to provide enlightenment. In fact, my new role at Hadassah only deepened my personal struggle. With greater responsibility for patients, I became more personally connected to them, and each new case seemed to present a new type of misfortune. My initial instinct at being exposed to so much suffering was just to give up on God. Why struggle? Why not simply abandon the idea of God, when so much evidence would seem to point to the impossibility of His existence? But despite all the suffering I was witnessing, perhaps even because of it, I was also aware of an element of the sacred that persisted throughout my patients' experiences. "I cannot prove its existence," Mahatma Gandhi wrote of the divine, "but what I can say is that the unanimous contradiction of the entire world will not weaken me in my faith that what I have heard is the voice of God. To me this voice is more real than my own existence." As a physician caring for children facing serious illness, I am granted access to intense, often tragic, but sometimes beautiful moments in people's lives. It is in these human interactions that I see that glimmer of the divine. Despite all of the terrible things I see, I also get to witness incredible moments: parents embracing and strengthening each other and then doing the same for their children, families refusing to surrender to despair. I am convinced that I am watching something sacred.

IN MY STRUGGLES WITH PHILOSOPHY and theology, I'm becoming increasingly interested in a school of thought called process theology. This is a theory that posits, through somewhat dense reasoning, that God does exist and is a force for good, but, for reasons we cannot understand, He is also limited. Although He has a will in this world and wishes only for good, there are certain things He cannot accomplish because they are beyond His control. The best-known proponent of this view might be Rabbi Harold Kushner, whose book *When Bad Things Happen to Good People* reaches a similar conclusion. It's a complicated theology, and as I struggle with it I do not find it completely satisfying, but it feels more right to me than either accepting a world with no God or a world where God actually allows (or wills!) children to die of terrible diseases. And, admittedly on a somewhat hubristic level, this is something I can relate to. Doctors are often accused of thinking they are godlike creatures (though at times it feels like this is what families expect of us, godlike feats), but in this respect process theology resonates with how I experience my role as a physician: I want only the best for my patients, I do my best for them, but sometimes it's just not possible to achieve the miracle they are hoping for.

. . .

ELISHEVA HAS BEEN MY PATIENT for a little more than a year. Fortunately, the muscle tumor in her arm had been detected before it had a chance to spread, and she has just completed her last course of planned chemotherapy. I would be seeing her today for one final meeting before transferring her to our follow-up clinic, where patients who have completed treatment are monitored over the years for signs of recurrence or long-term side effects of chemotherapy. Elisheva is from a Modern Orthodox Jewish family. She's in her early twenties and was just out of school and starting to discuss marriage with her boyfriend when she received her diagnosis (at which point he promptly disappeared from her life). She has an outsize personality and lights up any room she walks into with her big, toothy smile and laughing eyes. Through a difficult year of chemotherapy, surgery, and radiation, I only rarely saw her looking tired or down. For the most part she exuded positivity and was a beacon of cheerfulness, someone to whom staff and patients alike always seemed to be drawn.

I use these end-of-therapy meetings to reflect back on the achievement of having completed chemotherapy, to review what to expect in the follow-up clinic, and to discuss how to begin to get back to a "normal" life. The meeting with Elisheva is brief and straightforward, business as usual for me. She has always displayed great maturity, and I assume that if she has any concerns she will bring them up herself. I figure that at this point she must simply want to finish up, get out of here, and get on with her life.

As we wind down the meeting I conclude with my customary speech thanking her for letting me be a part of her care team. I hunch over my desk to write her (hopefully) last prescription for a minor antibiotic that she is still taking. But midway through the prescription I pause. I had recently traveled to Boston for a short course in palliative care, something I hadn't known that much about previously. Among the topics covered was the issue of spiritual support for patients. Oddly, though I had spent years preoccupied with my own theological musings, it hadn't occurred to me to ask about the spiritual challenges my patients, facing truly life-threatening situations, might be struggling with. Figuring that now is as good a time as any to test out some of the new ideas I had learned in Boston, I take a deep breath and feel my way forward.

"Elisheva," I say carefully, "I hope you'll forgive me for asking and please let me know if I've crossed a line, but I was wondering about how this whole experience has affected your sense of community and your belief system, especially as an observant Jew? Has anything changed for you?"

She is silent for a moment, and I look up just in time to see her burst into tears. It's the first time I have ever seen her cry. After a few minutes of quiet weeping, as I sit there feeling terrible and wondering what to do, Elisheva unleashes a torrent of spiritual angst. She describes her sense of alienation from her community, her worries that she is now "damaged goods" and will never marry, and that despite having undergone ovarian cryopreservation she still might never be able to have children. She asks repeatedly what she has done to deserve this. She worries that despite having done everything "right," as an observant Jew she has somehow angered God and brought this on herself.

I am mortified. A few minutes ago I had been so proud of our mutual accomplishments, of having successfully treated her cancer. But now that pride dissolves into despair, even panic, as I realize that I had neglected to address a critical aspect of Elisheva's care. I am sending off to long-term follow-up someone who is physically cured but who has been spiritually damaged. I wonder how I could have missed this in my interactions with her. She had always seemed so happy; perhaps I had just assumed that if anything had been troubling her spiritually, she would have consulted a rabbi from her community. She and I are so differently observant that I'm sure it would never have occurred to her to bring up her spiritual distress with me. For the same reason, it certainly never occurred to me to broach the subject with her. But more than that, I think that being attuned to the spiritual needs of our patients has simply been trained out of us as clinicians. I have no idea how to respond to Elisheva's outburst. Instead, I mumble some platitudes about it not being her fault, all the while knowing that my answer is completely inadequate and that fixing this sort of damage is beyond my skill set.

For much of history, religion and healing have been inextricably linked. Examples abound from across eras and cultures, ranging from the ancient Israelite priesthood to Native American shamans to Tibetan Buddhist healers (to name but a few examples). But in the modern era, spirituality and medicine seem to have not just been separated in the name of science but also to have become estranged. In the United States, my experience had been that a patient's spiritual needs in the hospital were always left to the chaplains. At no point in my medical training was I ever taught to address the spiritual needs of my patients; at no point was I even taught that it's an issue at all. We would do all we could medically for our patients, and then, once medicine had nothing left to offer, we would call in the chaplains. It sometimes felt as though the degree to which doctors consider spirituality to be important for patient care is inversely proportional to the likelihood of a cure. It was the rare but insightful clinician who would suggest a visit by the hospital chaplain to a patient who was not facing the real possibility of death.

In Israel, the concept of hospital chaplaincy barely exists, with just the earliest movement toward what is euphemistically being labeled "spiritual accompaniment" now starting to emerge. Ironically, this seems to be because religion is woven into the very fabric of the state, and Israelis both religious and secular seem to arrive at similar conclusions about spiritual support, albeit from opposite sides of the spectrum. Mention spiritual support in the hospital and the staff reacts as though you have trampled on the philosophical or religious dignity of anyone within earshot. Secular people are incensed that you would dare to drag a God who does not exist into the picture and that you would want to mix someone's private spiritual beliefs with science. Religious people are insulted that you would dare to undermine the authority of the spiritual leaders of their own communities. "It's none of your business," I've been told by our staff. "They have their own rabbi/imam/priest, and it's not your job to worry about that sort of thing."

Because religion is such a hot-button issue in Israel, Israelis seem to have a hard time discussing spirituality as something that can exist outside of organized religion. "You're so American," they say with disdain when I try to broach this subject. "That's such an American idea." This, of course, stings all the more because I am trying so hard to figure out how to fit into Israeli society, but it also strikes me as narrow-minded and self-defeating.

Regardless of how clinicians personally feel about spiritual matters, a fair amount of literature has emerged over the past few years suggesting that spiritual care should in fact be a routine part of medical care—certainly when dealing with patients facing potentially life-threatening illness. Adult patients, even those self-identifying as nonreligious, report that they want their spiritual needs explored. Adults who feel that their spiritual needs are being addressed say they feel better and are more satisfied with their care. The same evidence doesn't exist yet in pediatrics, probably because so few studies have been done. As it is, spirituality is relegated to the hinterlands in the world of medicine, and designing a study on the spiritual needs of children, who are considered a vulnerable research population, is tricky. Any research would have to take into account the developmental differences among children across a wide age range; a four-year-old's concept of spirituality and ability to discuss that concept is completely different from that of a nine-year-old or a fifteen-year-old. But given what we know about adults facing illness and how important spiritual needs are for them, it's worrying that we may be missing similar spiritual distress in children. From the few published studies that I've read, it does seem that many, if not most, children and young adults facing potentially life-threatening illness use spirituality and/or religion as a source of support and that the exploration of those needs could strengthen and enhance these coping mechanisms. And interestingly enough, some evidence suggests that a significant minority of sick children and young adults experience religion and spirituality via negative coping mechanisms; like Elisheva, they experience a sense of rejection, self-blame, and despair as a result of their beliefs. There can be no doubt that addressing the spiritual needs of sick children and young adults at risk of negative coping could have a positive impact on their well-being. For clinicians, knowing where and how to find more expert spiritual support should be a critical part of delivering complete care to our younger patients. Though we are not expected to be spiritual specialists, we all should be expected to have some skills as spiritual generalists. We should know how to ask basic questions to determine whether spiritual needs are being met and, if necessary, how to access the appropriate experts. I'm not a surgeon and would never be expected to perform an appendectomy, but as a pediatrician I am certainly expected to be able to identify a child with possible appendicitis and to call the surgeon. So it should be with spiritual needs. In Elisheva's case, while I may not have been the right person to manage her spiritual distress, I do think I was the person who should have picked up on it and been able to refer her to either a member of our hospital chaplaincy staff or a community leader who could have helped her. Instead, I missed it entirely and left her spiritually wounded.

WHILE THE MEDICAL WORLD DELIBERATELY keeps religious matters at arm's length, a few months into my practice at Hadassah I discover that the reverse is certainly not the case. One Thursday afternoon, as I'm finishing up in the clinic before the start of the weekend, I'm handed the phone to take a call from a man whose name is unfamiliar to me.

"Hello," I say. "This is Dr. Waldman."

"Yes?" he says, with a questioning tone, as though he is answering the phone and expects me to explain why I'm bothering him. There are a few moments of silence before I realize he isn't going to say anything else.

I try again. "Hi, yes, this is Dr. Waldman on the phone, pediatric oncology."

"Yes, Doctor." Same tone, followed by same silence.

"Um, you called me?" I say. "How can I help you?"

"Rabbi Perl wants to talk to you."

"Okay," I say, waiting for him to explain who Rabbi Perl is.

Long silence. "So," he finally says, "what number can he reach you at?"

"I'll be right here in the clinic until five or so," I say. "He can use the same number you called and just ask for me."

"And after five?"

"Well, he can try me here again any time after eight in the morning on Sunday, when the clinic opens again." There is no way I'm giving out my private cellphone number to some stranger, especially given the tone of this exchange. There's a very long silence.

"But if he wants to speak with you before then?" he asks insistently.

"I won't be on call again until Sunday morning, so if there's some medical emergency, it's best to go through the hospital operator to contact my colleague who will be on call Friday and Saturday."

There's another long silence, during which I get the distinct impression that he is baffled by me and by my response. I honestly feel the same way about him. It's as though there's some piece of this conversation that each of us is missing, or perhaps the two of us aren't even talking about the same thing.

"Okay," he finally says, sounding exasperated, and hangs up without so much as a goodbye.

One of the nurses, a Haredi woman, happens to be sitting next to me at the front desk throughout the phone call. She looks up, somewhat ominously, with one eyebrow rising under the stiff bangs of her wig.

"That was Perl's assistant?" she asks.

I shrug, annoyed by the whole thing. "So what? He gets special treatment? I have no idea who he is or what he wants. This guy doesn't even introduce himself properly, and I'm just supposed to hand out my personal phone number?"

"Be careful," she says. It's clear that she has considerable respect for this person, whoever he is. "It's a big deal that he's calling you, and it's worth it for you to be nice to him. He can make your career here." She doesn't explain further.

I don't hear from Rabbi Perl on Sunday, or for the rest of that week, but in asking around I do learn about him and the cultlike aura that surrounds him. It turns out that Rabbi Perl is one of *the* go-to sources for medical advice for most of Israel. He advises families on medically related issues ranging from which doctor to choose to which treatment or procedure to select for any specific illness. A recommendation from him can funnel all business for any given ailment through a particular clinician's office, or, more destructively, can direct all traffic *away* from a clinician, leading a practice and a career to wither. Perhaps because I have now become sensitized to it, I start noticing Perl's name cropping up in my dealings with my patients. Many of them, it turns out, seek his advice at every point throughout the treatment plan that we have worked out, even on issues that to me seem fairly straightforward. I discover that upon leaving my office after a consultation or treatment, many of them make a beeline for his office to report on what transpired and get his advice on how to proceed. And patients who arrive late for treatments will sometimes explain, with a shrug, that their appointment with Rabbi Perl ran long.

I find all of this quite horrifying, not to mention a bit insulting. Even more surprising to me is that this phenomenon is not limited to the observant population. Secular, and even anti-religious people often seek an audience with Perl, despite their disdain for anything that smacks of religion and despite the fact that he has had no medical training. One afternoon, sitting at a café in Tel Aviv, I mention this to a couple of friends, well-off secular Israelis. I express my surprise at and, I admit, even scorn for people who would seek medical advice, especially for life-threatening illness, from someone like Perl. I'm astonished when they interrupt me to say, "Perl? Of course! We saw him when we were about to have our first child! How else would we know who the best doctor would be for our needs?"

"But *everyone* wants the best doctor," I explode. "No one says, 'I'd like to see a mediocre doctor when I'm having my first child.' Or, 'I'm looking for a mediocre doctor to cure my child's cancer!' How does the rest of the world manage without Dr. Perl?"

They mumble something about how this is the system here, it's what's accepted, and that I'm just being an American. But I can't get my head around it, and we eventually change the topic.

The first time I actually meet Rabbi Perl it's by chance, when he stops by the department to talk with Mickey. We are introduced, and I, of course, address him cordially and perhaps even, I'm embarrassed to admit, with some deference. There is no formal interview, but I know that Mickey later talks me up to him, and that he's impressed by the fact that I have connections to a major cancer center back in the United States. Despite how I feel about the whole thing, I confess to experiencing some small pleasure when I realize that, sometime after our conversation, Perl has begun referring patients, especially those with progressive disease, to me. I subsequently discover that he isn't the only rabbi in Israel to whom people go for medical refer-rals and advice. Though there is no evidence whatsoever that their recommendations lead to better treatment, the entire country seems convinced that regardless of your own religious background, consulting these guys is just the way it's done. Perl sometimes calls me himself, and I take his calls seriously, telling myself that it's for my patients' sake that I'm going along with all this, so that they can feel confident that they are getting the best care possible. But the truth is that some part of me, the part that is trying to find my place in Israeli society, is pleased at receiv-ing Perl's imprimatur. I am starting to understand the degree to which religion permeates all aspects of society here, and accom-modating Rabbi Perl seems to be a part of locating myself within that society.

HOW IRONIC IT IS that a medical system that has so delib-erately removed religion and spirituality from our consideration in matters of patient care is in so many ways in thrall to rab-bis with no formal medical training. When I stand in the fam-ily area of our department, in front of the floor-to-ceiling glass windows looking out onto the biblical landscape that figures so prominently in the Scriptures of Jews, Muslims, and Christians, it seems to me so obvious and so natural that here of all places we should recognize the necessity of addressing spiritual needs and physical needs together, as part of a holistic approach to patient care.

On the other hand, religion and spirituality are incredibly complicated here, to the point where their external trappings have become almost tribal symbols, public indicators that allow for immediate religious and political classification. For men, for example, a round black hat and long black coat, *payos,* and a long beard signal a Haredi—politically conservative, possibly anti-Zionist. Casual khaki trousers, a short-sleeved shirt, and a knitted *kippah* indicate someone who is Modern Orthodox, Zionistic, and most likely politically conservative. But a much larger knitted *kippah* on someone similarly garbed, and with perhaps some indication of *payos* and a pistol tucked into the waistband of his pants, proclaims that this person most likely lives in a settlement somewhere on the West Bank and fully intends to remain there, come what may. And those are just the Ashkenazim. Mizrachim (Jews originally from North Africa, the Middle East, and other parts of the former Ottoman Empire) have their own categories of observance and accompanying modes of dress. These feel like stereotypes, but the code is undeniably there, and I am just learning how to read it.

My own level of observance is something that many of my colleagues find confusing. Although I do not wear a *kippah* on a daily basis, I am somewhat observant. I'm not sure how many of them are familiar with the principles of Conservative Judaism, with which I nominally identify; the Masorti (Conservative) movement in Israel is passionate but small. I'm also not shy about my leftward political leanings, which puzzle my colleagues even more. "How can you be religious but also be left-wing?" I am frequently asked. Orthodox friends and colleagues dismiss my claims to observance, as well as my politics, as being mushy and confused: I'm not *really* observant, they say, and I'm too new to the country to understand the politics. I'm still too American, they claim.

What I find particularly interesting is how connected to religious and holiday traditions many of my militantly secular friends in Tel Aviv are—most likely because the Sabbath and Jewish holidays are also part of the national culture, and because the Bible is our national literature. To my mind, any Jew in the United States possessing the level of observance and knowledge of Judaism and Jewish history of the average self-identified secular Israeli would be considered a Conservative Jew. But in Israel the divide between the religious and the secular is about much more than levels of observance. Here economics, politics, and sociology all find their way into the religious mix. On some level I can understand why my colleagues at Hadassah shy away from making room for religion and spirituality in the care of our patients.

But where does that leave Elisheva, who was clearly too uncomfortable with what she was feeling to consult with her community's religious authorities during her months of treatment? From time to time when she comes for appointments in the follow-up clinic, she stops by my office for a quick hello. I wonder what spiritual scar tissue may still be knotting up her soul and I wonder if, had I been more attuned to her spiritual needs, I would have been able to help with that aspect of her care and send her on her way better prepared to move forward with her life. I can't help but feel that in that respect I failed her.

EVEN AS OUR DEPARTMENT DOES ITS BEST to avoid getting involved in the spiritual care of our patients, and whether we want to acknowledge it or not, the very nature of our work involves spirituality. Particularly when it comes to end-of-life issues, there are many moments when, if you are paying attention, this manifests itself quite clearly.

After a long illness marked by remissions and recurrences, eight-year-old Naama is now spending her final days in our department; she's mostly unconscious but is still getting medication for management of pain and anxiety. I duck into her room now and then to monitor her clinical status and to make sure she is comfortable. These are critical hours, not just for our patients but also for their family members. A sudden cry of pain from a dying patient, or a seizure, or even just a disturbing moan might linger more painfully in the memories of parents and siblings than almost anything the child had gone through during her course of treatment. The nurses and I want to be sure that we can respond as quickly as possible to any changes in Naama's condition.

Even though it's the middle of the day, the room is dark. The window shades have been pulled down, and in the dim light from a bedside lamp I can just make out that Naama's breathing is slowing, the muscles of her face relaxing as death approaches. The room is crowded, full of extended family. It feels stuffy, and the air is sour from the bodies of so many people who have been holding this vigil for so many hours. But there is also an unmistakable sense of energy, purpose, and love in that room, and I feel it enveloping me as well. Naama's family are Bratslaver Hasidim (a Hasidic sect that is particularly focused on mysticism), and as I crouch at Naama's bedside to check her breathing, they began to sing, all of their voices joined together. I find myself simultaneously focused on her breathing and their singing. It's a song associated with Rabbi Nachman, the sect's founding rabbi: *The whole world is a very narrow bridge, and the main thing is to have no fear at all.*

AS I BEGIN TO RECOGNIZE the extent to which religious personalities and rulings influence Israeli society, I also gain first-hand experience with another (if not *the* other) force that exerts considerable influence on all aspects of life in Israel: the military. In Israel, military service is considered a major milestone (except for the Haredim, most of whom avail themselves of the controversial exemption for full-time Torah students, and the Arabs, who are exempt but who may volunteer for certain types of service). But any young person who has been diagnosed with cancer, no matter how far in the distant past this may have occurred, is exempt from the draft. They may choose to volunteer, but even then they're barred from joining a combat unit for fear that some undetected damage or weakness will manifest itself under the stress of training or, worse, during actual combat. Because military service is such a point of honor and pride in Israel, some of the adolescent boys we treat seem to take this harder than they take the cancer diagnosis itself. Young men who had been preparing themselves to try out for the toughest units suddenly find that the primary focus of their teenage identity is now gone. Their friends report for induction and these kids remain at home, listening to stories each weekend from the new recruits about exploits in which they will never get to take part and enviously eyeing sharp-looking uniforms and unit insignia. They can and do volunteer for noncombat positions, and many of our former patients proudly return to Hadassah after their induction to show themselves off to us in their own uniforms.

I got an unexpected and quite moving look into the world of noncombat volunteers in the Israeli army when I myself was drafted a little more than a year after making aliyah. Though I am way past the cutoff age for military service for men who make aliyah, the IDF does make an exception for physicians, whose skills remain in demand even as we enter middle age. I had figured I might be assigned to take a first-aid course for perhaps a month or two, so that I could help care for the reservists who periodically get called up from their civilian lives to do their "peacetime" military service. I was even sort of looking forward to this as a way of making an admittedly minor contribution to the IDF at little or no risk to myself. What American Jewish adolescent boy doesn't fantasize at some point about serving in the IDF? My brother had actually volunteered and served in an Israeli combat unit after college, and I was looking forward to getting my own small taste of army life. To my surprise, I was told at my first meeting at the draft center that I was being sent to combat medical officers' school, after which I was to spend a year in a combat unit. The officer in charge delivered this news to me with a bright and excited smile, as though she were announcing that I had won the lottery.

"Just think," she said, "we can arrange for you to be in the same unit that your brother was in! Start a family tradition! How great!"

I wasn't sure it was great at all. Eighteen months seemed like a long time to take off from being an oncologist. And, more to the point, fantasizing about serving in the IDF was one thing. Actually dodging bullets was quite another. I drove home shaking from a rush of adrenaline and fear.

After some backroom negotiations over the course of the next few days and some string-pulling by Hadassah colleagues connected with the army, it was agreed that I would complete the full five-month medical officers' course but that I would then have the option of signing on for at least a year of combat duty or going straight into the reserves. It was a pretty good deal. Five months away from oncology still seemed like a long time, but the course sounded interesting and I would end up being inducted into the IDF as an officer, which meant I would achieve the important goal of outranking my brother.

When call-up day arrived I was nervous, having been told only to pack lightly and show up at a certain place and time. I dressed in jeans and a T-shirt, and took enough clothes for a week, not sure what to expect. The only thing I knew about basic training was what I'd seen in Stanley Kubrick's *Full Metal Jacket.* I tried to brace myself for the IDF's version, which I was sure was going to be even worse. In the paved lot outside the induction center, proud and tearful parents embraced their teenagers, who tried to act brave in front of their family and friends. Every few minutes a loudspeaker would call out a bunch of names, and another group would say their goodbyes and file into a waiting bus that, once full, would rumble off into the unknown. Eventually my name was called, and I climbed onto a bus crammed with rowdy, nervous, and hormonal young men and women, wondering what I had gotten myself into. It turned out that our destination was a building just a couple hundred yards away. It would have been easily walkable, and this was my first experience of how the army appears to make a special point of taking a simple task and making it infinitely and needlessly more complex. We left the bus, crossed a parking lot, and headed toward a one-story, featureless gray building. Entering the camp truly felt like entering a different universe, a parallel Israel that exists in plain sight but is also hidden. I'd had an inkling of this world from hearing my brother talk about his own enlistment. As we filed into the induction center I was aware that I had almost mysteriously passed from one world to another, from civilian to soldier.

Inside, the concrete floors and corrugated steel walls gave the whole thing the appearance of a maze. We moved along in assembly-line fashion, passing from station to station. At one window we had our photos taken, at another ID cards were spit out of a laminating machine, at yet another uniforms and boots were thrust at us. At one particularly disturbing station we received injections that were tersely described as "vaccines" (though I could have sworn I was up to date with mine), and then had tissue swabbed from the insides of our mouths and stored for DNA analysis. I wondered how many of the kids realized that this DNA banking was intended to facilitate the identification of our remains should we ever be blown to bits or mangled beyond recognition. The thought was not comforting.

About an hour after we'd entered the building we were disgorged from its opposite side, now in uniform and carrying army kit bags full of gear. At least we were starting to look like soldiers. We were then separated into groups and herded into a small auditorium, where we were told to sit down and wait. I took the opportunity to look around the room and was concerned at not seeing anyone else who looked even close to my age. Where were the other medical inductees? Doctors do their medical service in the army after they have completed medical school, so they don't look like the average eighteen-year-old recruit, and the kids around me looked like, well, kids. As I started to really pay attention to the youngsters, I began to notice other things that seemed a bit strange. Some of the boys were obviously limping, some were severely cross-eyed with thick glasses, and others moved, spoke, or otherwise behaved in ways that were slightly off, suggestive of physical or neurological limitations. I wondered why I had been placed with them. I even began to worry that my assignment had been changed without my knowledge. But this was the great and mighty IDF, so I figured the army must have their reasons and that I'd meet up with my fellow medical inductees later.

An officer strode in and grabbed the podium. He appeared to be in his seventies, wore the rumpled fatigues of a reservist, and looked like he would be more at home alongside a pool in Florida, bragging about his grandchildren. He beamed, wrinkles forming at the corners of his eyes as he surveyed the room.

"I am so proud of you all!" he exclaimed.

Okay, I thought, I'm pretty proud also. I'm into this.

"Really!" he continued, even more emphatically. "I am so proud of each and every one of you and the amazing commitment you are showing to your country today!"

I was still in agreement, still pretty proud of myself, but his exuberance seemed a bit much. And he clearly wasn't done.

"Each of you has overcome so much already, so many challenges. Sicknesses, accidents. And yet you have volunteered to do what you can to help your country. *Kol ha-kavod!* We honor you!"

I now realized why the kids in this room seemed to be a bit off: they had all been exempted from military service for physical or psychological reasons and had volunteered anyway, for noncombat positions. I had drifted into the wrong auditorium. When we were eventually directed into a much larger area where groups of soldiers were gathering, I managed to locate the group of medical inductees and join them. As we waited around for our next instructions, I reflected on how much I admired those boys who had already overcome so much in their lives and were now determined to serve in the IDF in whatever way they could. It made me realize yet again how big a part military service played in determining one's societal worth in Israel, and why so many of the teenage boys that I treated made such a point of coming back to visit us once they were in uniform. In the future, when I would have to tell a teenage patient that because of his cancer he would no longer be eligible for combat service, I would be sure to tell him that I'd personally seen how much the IDF values its noncombat volunteers.

Before we actually started basic training, we were all formally sworn in as members of the IDF, our hands on military-issue Bibles. It was the summer of 2008, and on this day Hezbollah was transferring to Israel the bodies of two soldiers who had been killed back in 2006, in the attack that had sparked that summer's war in Lebanon. The mood in the camp that day was somber, and before swearing in the new recruits, the commander of the base broadcast over the loudspeakers a statement from the IDF chief of staff. It was a painful day, he said, but also a day to remember that just as all soldiers swear an oath to the State of Israel, so the State of Israel swears to its soldiers that no matter what happens, we will always be brought home. It was a sobering but proud moment for me. This was the courageous and compassionate Israel that I had admired from afar as I was growing up. Even more than when I made aliyah, I was filled with a sense of purpose and brotherhood as I now became an Israeli.

At the conclusion of the five-month medical training course I elected to bypass active duty and entered the reserves, which meant being periodically summoned from my civilian life to do a few weeks of military service a year and being available for call-up should a war break out. In the reserves, my duties ranged from fairly boring clinic work to practice drills for wartime to more interesting stints accompanying combat units to more remote bases. Upon my return to Hadassah, there was no question that I was treated differently by my colleagues—less like some clueless American and more like an Israeli who had made a commitment to his country. Getting that stamp of approval from Rabbi Perl, admiring my IDF rank tags—with these I began to feel the sense of belonging that I had been searching for.

8

Honey from Gaza

I T IS EARLY JANUARY 2009, and we are in the midst of the latest outbreak of hostilities between Israel and Hamas in Gaza. The goal of Operation Cast Lead, as the Israeli government calls it, is to halt the barrage of rockets that Hamas has been firing into Israel and that have been landing in civilian areas along Israel's border with Gaza. The department feels haunted. Not by the ghosts of former patients but, rather, by the living, by staff and patients who walk the halls as if uncertain of their place in this shifting world. On the first day of Israel's ground incursion into Gaza, I examine Ahmad, a sixteen-year-old Arab boy from East Jerusalem with a massive bone tumor in his shoulder that has been growing larger despite chemotherapy. Perched on the edge of the exam table, he pulls off his shirt as I stand in front of him. Around his neck hangs a gold-colored medallion in the shape of what, back in 1922, the League of Nations christened Mandatory Palestine. Nowadays, there are those who refer to this landmass as "greater Israel" and others who call it, simply, "Palestine." Ahmad's medallion is covered in the black, green, and red stripes of the Palestinian flag, so it's not hard to figure out where his politics lie.

I try to focus on the huge, misshapen tumor protruding from Ahmad's shoulder. But the medallion, a glimmering statement of more extreme Palestinian aspirations, distracts me. I've noticed it before, but now, with the war, it seems more deliberate. The more I try to ignore it, not to think about the message it is intended to send to people like me, the more I am distracted. I gently probe the tumor with my fingertips as I silently calculate its rate of growth and how much longer this young man has to live. Ahmad keeps his head down, only once briefly looking up at me with pained eyes that bore into mine out of a gray, emaciated face. What can he be thinking? Out there in his neighborhood he is a young Palestinian, struggling with his people's aspirations. In here, though neither of us has openly acknowledged it yet, he is dying. Is his glance a plea for my help? Is it suspicion and anger at my failure to cure him? Or is it simply resignation, an acknowledgment that despite my best efforts and his stoicism during months of treatment, he knows he is dying. I am not sure I want to know the answer.

I ask Ahmad if he needs pain medication, trying to focus on the things I can control. But inside I am sick and angry at my inability to do anything more for him. I ridicule myself for behaving as though the sum total of his problems can be solved with a few morphine pills.

When I'm finished with Ahmad, I head for my next patient, and in the corridor I run into Tal and her mother. Tal is a one-year-old who has been recently diagnosed with a brain tumor. She also happens to live near Sderot, an Israeli town just a mile or so from the border with Gaza that has borne the brunt of countless rocket and mortar attacks by Hamas over the past several years. Not long after Tal's initial diagnosis I was talking with her mother when she suddenly burst into tears. Isn't it hard enough to raise a child under constant fear of rocket fire, she sobbed, now we've got to fight her cancer at the same time? I just stood there, at a complete loss for words. Now I bend over and give Tal a tickle, eliciting a squeal. How's everything? I ask her mother. The question is deliberately nonspecific. Am I asking how a one-year-old is coping with her chemotherapy? How she and her family are handling going to sleep every night in an underground shelter as they listen to the sounds of rocket fire just across the fields? I don't know which question would be more impossible to answer. Tal's mother understands. "Okay," she whispers, but her bloodshot eyes give a very different reply.

Later that same day I am on rounds with my team when my cellphone rings. It's my commanding officer in the reserves. He tells me to organize my gear when I get home, as our unit will surely be called up if the conflict spreads. I hang up and return to rounds, but now my mind is racing. I try to focus on the resident presenting the patient at hand: overnight vital signs, relevant lab values, major changes. I try to lead the discussion, make a few teaching points, develop a treatment plan for the day. But a part of my mind has already fled the scene, trying to remember where I left my army kit bag, if my boots are with it, whether I have enough clean socks. This is my first potential call-up to active duty. As I check chemotherapy orders I wonder, What does one pack for a war?

The child-friendly atmosphere that we work so hard to promote in our department—the clowns, the arts and crafts, the music, and the videogames—is now no more than a veneer of pleasantness that barely covers the turbulent undercurrents. In every patient's room, in every treatment area, the television broadcasts nothing but images of Israeli air strikes on Gaza and Hamas rockets falling on Israeli towns. At the front desk, the department secretary tries to keep a smile on as she arranges patients' appointments while staying glued to her radio. Her husband got a call to join his army unit at three o'clock in the morning. He quickly grabbed his gear and left, unable, of course, to tell her exactly where he was going or when he would return.

Two days later I hear that a doctor whom I had met during our army training course and with whom I'd become friends has been killed in the fighting. I am horrified, but after some frantic checking I discover that it was actually another reserve medical officer in his unit who has been killed. Uncomfortable relief washes over me. A doctor who only a week ago was treating patients in his office is now a dead soldier. I struggle to assimilate this, to figure out who I am in this surreal environment: doctor? soldier? Israeli? American? Can I be all of the above?

While on my rounds I run into Musa in the hall and give him a high five. Musa is a ten-year-old boy from Gaza who had the great misfortune to be diagnosed with leukemia about a week before this current round of fighting began. Because he has an uncle who lives not far from Jerusalem, in one of the Palestinian-controlled areas in the West Bank, his family initially obtained a pass from the Israeli government to leave their home in Gaza and come to Hadassah for Musa's treatment, with the expectation that they would be able to obtain another pass to stay with the uncle when Musa was ready to have his chemotherapy on an outpatient basis. Musa responded well to his initial inpatient chemotherapy, and he is now ready to be discharged and come in just for outpatient treatments. But when the fighting broke out, the government stopped issuing passes to and from the Palestinian-controlled areas in the West Bank, and so Musa and his mother are stuck here, unable to stay with the uncle while Musa gets his chemotherapy. We keep him admitted, though there is no medical reason for him to be here, so that at least he has a bed and he and his mother get meal trays while we wait to see how things end. As my colleagues and I do our rounds in the mornings we often run into Musa strolling the halls, smiling at everyone and giving out high fives. He reminds me of the Tom Hanks character in the movie *The Terminal,* trapped in political/

administrative limbo. But this isn't a movie, and there is nothing funny about his situation.

My final visit of the day is to a child in our hospice room. It is evening, and through the picture windows at the end of the hall I can see lights twinkling in the Arab village across the valley. I remind myself to call friends in Tel Aviv with whom I've made dinner plans, to let them know I'm running a bit late. I enter the room, smile, and in my limited Arabic greet the father of this young Palestinian boy who doesn't have very much longer to live. Propped up in the bed, bloated from steroids, and barely responsive, Jamil had been managed as an outpatient for some time, but his inoperable brain tumor has become too much for his parents to bear alone, so they have brought him to Hadassah for his final days.

I give Jamil's arm a squeeze and say hello, though at this point I'm not certain that he hears me; he is already breathing the wet, slow breaths that indicate death is approaching. The nurse who would normally assist with translation is busy, so I sit at Jamil's bedside, next to his father, resting a hand on his arm, trying to convey in body language what I cannot verbalize.

We sit in silence, watching the slow rise and fall of Jamil's chest and listening to the soft drone of the news in Arabic coming from the television above our heads. After a few moments I glance up. The television is tuned to a Palestinian station, and the images are of the damage the Israeli air strikes are doing in Gaza—buildings destroyed, children injured, parents crying. I look back down at Jamil as I massage his swollen arm and avoid making eye contact with his father, wondering what I'd say if I were able to communicate with him in Arabic.

ONE WEEKEND DURING THE CONFLICT, a group of American and European expats organize a get-together on the beach in Tel Aviv. Despite the chill wind off the ocean and overcast skies, we come together because none of us has family close by, and with so much violence and uncertainty in the air we turn to each other for support, an ad hoc family of idealists. Some people bring large Israeli flags, in keeping with the spirit of patriotism and solidarity with the troops. As we mill around chatting and catching up, a squad of attack helicopters sweeps by overhead, flying southward. They are close enough that we can make out the pilots' faces, and as we wave our flags they dip and wiggle their copters in acknowledgment. I am struck by the thought that in just a few minutes these pilots will be over Gaza, delivering their payloads—hopefully onto a bunch of Hamas fighters, but quite possibly onto some unsuspecting civilians who are in the wrong place at the wrong time.

As the helicopter gunships head off, one of the Americans in the group puffs out his chest and declares that he has absolutely no qualms about the military action in Gaza, adding that the situation has complete moral clarity for him and that he has never felt more certain about anything in his life. The woman next to him rolls her eyes. I am baffled by his certainty. I support our troops and the mission of the State of Israel to protect its citizens—I'm still a soldier on standby myself. But our military intelligence is not infallible, and the scenes on television of carnage at a building that was once a school or at a marketplace are very hard to see. And despite our intention to strike back only at Hamas's military infrastructure in order to degrade their ability to threaten us, there is, intentional or not, an inevitable and undeniable element of collective punishment as everyone in Gaza suffers.

It's also hard to leave all this outside the hospital. On my first day back at Hadassah after my officer training, the mothers of two Palestinian children being treated in our clinic greet me warmly. "Where have you been?" they exclaim. I panic. Do I tell them that I've been off in the army? The same army that routinely appears in their villages in the middle of the night, looking for terrorists? Or do I make up some lie about where I've spent the past five months? I take a deep breath and tell them that I've been in a medical training course in the army. I had been so proud of what I'd been doing, even enjoying the training and looking forward to my first deployment in the reserves, so I am annoyed with myself when I feel my face flush with embarrassment. The women's faces fall for an instant. But then, barely missing a beat, one of them looks up at me, manages a small smile, and says, "We wish there were more people like you in the army. Maybe things would be different then."

THE BROADER REPERCUSSIONS of the Gaza incursion begin to ripple through our department. Though Israel's fight is with the more radical Hamas-led government in Gaza, the Fatah-led government in the PA, with which Israel has developed a modicum of cooperation over the years, must worry about its own political survival and answer to its constituents. A weakening of Hamas at Israel's hands may be beneficial to Fatah (which was ejected from Gaza by Hamas in a spasm of bloody violence in 2007), but the PA leadership apparently feels that it cannot be seen as implicitly endorsing any Israeli attacks on any Palestinians. And so one Thursday afternoon, as the fighting draws to a close, the PA announces with no warning that effective immediately it will no longer allow Palestinians to seek medical treatment in Israel. In this way they will not be opening themselves up to charges that they are collaborating in any way at all with the "enemy." But the only losers here are going to be thousands of sick Palestinians; the level of care they get in Israeli hospitals is for the most part not available in the West Bank. Because this announcement comes just as the weekend is starting, there is no time for our staff to discuss what will happen if the PA actually follows through and our patients are suddenly cut off from their radiation and chemotherapy treatments. Many of my colleagues shrug as we head out the door, either dismissing the PA's announcement as hollow political posturing or saying that if it does happen it's an internal Palestinian matter that they should be left to deal with themselves.

I can't imagine that the PA would actually forbid sick people to continue receiving medical care in Israel. I share what's been going on with friends at a café in Tel Aviv the next morning, only to find that nobody believes me. They all assume that I either misunderstood what the PA said or that I'm exaggerating. Their response stings. The cultural and political bubble that is Tel Aviv can often make people here feel as disconnected from Hadassah and the rest of Jerusalem as from the Palestinian towns beyond the Green Line. Though I love the city and the fact that its overwhelmingly liberal politics align with my own hopes for Israel's future, at times it's too easy in Tel Aviv to forget the realities of our situation with the Palestinians and the PA.

At the very least, I think to myself when I return to my apartment, the PA will surely make an exception for people being treated for cancer—not to mention children being treated for cancer. They've got excellent and devoted doctors over there, too, and they know the consequences of halting a patient's course of radiation therapy or chemotherapy, or the problems that could arise in redirecting patients to hospitals in Egypt or Jordan without their medical charts to accompany them. But when I return to Hadassah on Sunday morning, we quickly realize that no Palestinian patients are showing up for their appointments. There's not much to say; we are all just quietly devastated.

Operation Cast Lead is officially over on January 18, but the PA does not revoke its order. Weeks go by. A slight trickle of Palestinian patients begins to appear, as the few whose families have the right connections or enough money for a bribe manage to get permission to cross the checkpoints and come back for their treatments. But most of our patients simply disappear. We hear from a few families here and there. Some have gone to Egypt or Jordan for treatment, and some have managed, somehow, to get a few basic medications at home. But for the most part there is silence. It is many months before Palestinian patients start to appear at Hadassah in their former numbers, when the PA decides that their point has been made and that referrals may resume. Most of the children who turn up when the restrictions are lifted are new patients; only a handful of our old patients are among them. It isn't clear how many of those who do not return have completed their treatment elsewhere, how many are continuing to get treatment abroad, and how many have simply died. Of the children who do return, some seem to be doing fine despite the disruption, others return with relapsed disease, and still more end up relapsing later on. I don't know if the disruption in therapy is what led to the recurrences or if those kids just had fundamentally aggressive cancers that would have relapsed anyway. We will never be able to answer that terrible question. I know that their families will be wondering about this forever. I doubt the PA has given it any thought.

It's during this period that I find my interest in pediatric palliative care growing. Though many assume that palliative care refers to hospice and end-of-life care (and, indeed, these do fall under the purview of palliative care practitioners), in its modern incarnation pediatric palliative care is much broader in scope: it is a holistic approach to providing support for children facing potentially life-threatening illness and for their families. I've always been interested in the more humanities-oriented aspects of medicine. I can probably trace this as far back as my undergraduate interest in theology. But through my work at Hadassah I've become increasingly interested in how we guide patients and their families through difficult decision making—not just at the end of life but also when making major decisions during a child's therapy that may have serious implications for what his or her life will look like in the future.

I remember one of my fellow residents telling me years earlier why she had decided against going into pediatric oncology. It's all just protocols, she said. You plug a child with a given diagnosis into a treatment plan and simply follow the prescribed pathway. But that wasn't my experience. I realized pretty quickly, even as a fellow in oncology, that things tend not to be so clearcut. And here in Israel, as a more senior physician, I continually experience the complexities of decisions that clinicians, patients, and families must make together. When, for example, is it okay to "wiggle" the timing of treatments? Most protocols dictate very specific timing. But what if an important family event, such as a wedding or a summer trip, is coming up that the treatment would interfere with? Is it okay to delay treatments for something like that? Does the decision depend on what we think the actual chances of the patient's survival are? (And who really makes that determination?) Other examples might be more subtle, such as when we recommend surgery to remove a tumor and when we instead rely on radiation therapy. That may seem straightforward, but the evidence isn't always definitive, and the decision may also depend on such factors as the location of the tumor and how much damage each treatment might cause. Finally, in situations where standard therapies have failed, there are always questions about whether to try experimental therapies, weighing the risks of those therapies against the potential benefits—all of which often feels simply like educated guesswork. When those therapies are available only abroad, an additional layer of complexity is introduced. When do you recommend that parents use all their savings and uproot themselves and the rest of their family to take their child abroad for a high-risk therapy? And how do you guide a family for whom that is not an option, understanding that remaining in Israel means going down a path toward palliation and death?

In order to deepen my understanding of palliative care, I decide to return to the United States in 2010 for an intensive two-week course at Boston Children's Hospital, with the expectation that what I learn there will help me take better care of my patients at Hadassah. But the course only whets my appetite to learn more. I learn a lot about palliative care, about having more effective conversations with patients, about symptom manage- ment, and, more concretely, about some of the practical aspects of developing a program. But most of all I learn that there is an entire field of study developing around palliative care. Since 2008 it has been recognized in the United States as a separate medical subspecialty, with its own training programs and separate board certification. In Boston I discover people speaking a language that makes sense to me, one for which I feel I have been search- ing for years. I'm hooked, and in 2011 I apply for and am accepted to a yearlong fellowship program at Boston Children's to develop an expertise in pediatric palliative care, at the end of which I will be eligible to take the board certification exam to be a pediatric palliative care specialist. My colleagues at Hadassah greet the idea warily. What will you really gain from this? they ask. And to uproot yourself yet again? Most of them, I'm certain, think that once I've become settled back in America, I won't want to return to Israel when the fellowship ends. And although I assure them that I will be back (Hadassah has promised to hold my position for me), I admit to myself that a part of me is not so sure.

To be honest, I believe that this course of study will make me a better clinician at Hadassah, but it also comes at a point when I feel that I need a bit of distance from my life in Israel. I need to think about what sort of progress I've made over the past five years in figuring out who I am and where I belong. I've certainly grown as a doctor and as a person, but where I truly belong is still an open question. I've become aware of the fact that now, when I spend time in America, I actually feel more like an Israeli. I hold myself with a little more of a swagger. I speak somewhat more abrasively. For all of the annoyance I feel at the lack of formality and professional boundaries in Israel, when I'm in America I find myself missing the warmth and sense of community that accompanies it. And yet when I'm in Israel, I still feel like I'm walking around with a sign on my back that screams AMERICAN. I'm sure that plenty of American immigrants feel the same way, but the ones whom I know all seem to be comfortable with this duality—some of them actually enjoy it. I don't know why I don't. Perhaps spending this year away will help me figure this out.

The feeling that I need to spend some time away from Israel comes as a bit of a surprise to me. I had made aliyah in the firm belief that I was coming "home." I was positive that becoming part of this great liberal Zionist project, helping to contribute to the success of the national experiment to create a country whose goal is to be, as the prophet Isaiah says, "a light unto the nations," would give my life meaning and purpose. It took no time for me to realize how naive I was. I have become Israeli, but I'm still American. I'm both religious and secular. On some issues I side with the political left and on others with the political right. Which means that there isn't any one community in Israel in which I feel completely at home. The irony of my situation does not escape me.

I tell myself that I am going to Boston because I want to become proficient in pediatric palliative care, that the experience will be invaluable in advancing my career in Israel. Fellowships in this emerging field are still few and far between, and the program at Boston Children's is a prestigious one, led by Dr. Joanne Wolfe, the same doctor whose work on the suffering of dying children I had read at the outset of my medical training in 2000. With the training I receive there, I will be able to return to Israel as an expert (maybe even *the* expert) in pediatric palliative care. To change the shape of healthcare delivery for seriously ill children in Israel, in the West Bank, and in Gaza—and perhaps even across the region—now that would be the realization of my Zionist dream! But the truth is that as I make plans to return to Boston, I feel defeated. I am not at all sure what I will end up doing with the fellowship, not at all sure that I will even return to Israel when it ends. I worry that this fellowship is just a way to extricate myself from a complicated situation in Israel that I lack the maturity or the will to deal with, or that it's simply the latest example of my inability to "settle down." Hedging my bets, I place my belongings in storage and give up my apartment by the sea.

The day before I'm scheduled to leave for Boston happens to be the day that Gilad Shalit, the Israeli soldier taken prisoner by Hamas in June 2006, is released. Hearing the news in Guatemala about the fighting that had broken out between Hamas and Israel during that period was one of the triggers for my decision to move to Israel. That I'm leaving Israel during an event that will hopefully bring a sense of closure to that difficult time also strikes me as ironic.

The weeks leading up to Shalit's release—which was conditioned on the release from Israel of more than a thousand mostly Palestinian and Israeli Arab prisoners—are tense and emotional ones in Israel, marked by protests and acrimony. Though, of course, everyone wants to see Shalit back home alive, many worry that negotiating for the release of a kidnapped soldier will only create further incentive for more kidnappings by terrorists. Even among those who support the negotiations between Israel and Hamas, many balk at the extraordinarily high price being demanded for the release of just one person. Among the prisoners slated for release are many who have perpetrated violent crimes against Israelis, which, of course, causes great anguish among surviving relatives of the victims. For weeks Israel is consumed by angry debates, and the country's distress is palpable and inescapable. When the deal with Hamas is announced, only one thing is certain: no one is completely happy about it. But, as I learned at my own swearing-in ceremony, one of the principles upon which Israel prides itself is that no captured soldier—living or dead—will ever be abandoned. At the very least, Shalit's return should mark the end of a difficult chapter.

I arrive at Hadassah that morning planning to say my good-

byes to the staff and patients and then leave. I hate long farewells, and I had briefly considered slipping away without saying
a word to anyone. But it turns out that I needn't have worried
about being the uncomfortable focus of everyone's good wishes.
All attention is centered on the newscasters reporting on the
prisoner exchange scheduled for later that morning. Everyone
wonders what sort of shape Shalit is in, and whether Hamas or
some lone extremists might not attempt some last-minute sabo-
tage. As the morning proceeds the anxiety mounts.

As part of the security preparations surrounding the exchange, Israel's border with Gaza has been sealed. Often when
the borders are closed for security reasons, families with medical passes can still cross into Israel. But what's happening today
is unprecedented and, given the degree of tension, we assume
that none of our patients from Gaza will be arriving for their
regularly scheduled appointments. Indeed, there are noticeably
fewer patients than usual in the waiting areas today. As I walk
down the hallway and pass all the television sets broadcasting
live feeds from the Gaza border, waiting for Shalit to appear, I'm
reminded of the tension that filled our department three years
earlier, during Operation Cast Lead.

It turns out to be harder to leave than I thought it would be.
I wander through the clinic and the inpatient ward, saying my
goodbyes, watching everyone busy at work. I'm excited about
what awaits me in Boston, but I'm also sad to be leaving this
wonderful department and to be leaving my parents and siblings
(my brother and my parents recently made aliyah and are now
living in Tel Aviv). As I watch the drama unfold on the television
screens, I again feel ashamed. At this time of great national angst,
when—for however brief a moment—all Israelis are united, I am
leaving.

The time passes slowly. By late morning the actual prisoner
exchange begins. Doctors, nurses, patients, and their families are
silently riveted to the television sets. Suddenly, there's a com-
motion down the hall. A dozen or so people—our patients from

Gaza and their families—have burst from the elevators and are marching happily toward the center of the clinic. A number of them carry large trays covered in thick plastic wrap. *"Mabrouk! Mabrouk!"* they cry. "Blessings!" Placing their trays on the counter, they peel back the sheets of plastic to reveal an assortment of baklava, a syrupy sticky-sweet pastry made of delicately layered phyllo dough and nuts that have been saturated in honey. I generally love this sweet dessert, though after one bite I always remember why it is so often consumed along with dark, bitter Turkish coffee. It's not unusual for families to bring gifts to our department to celebrate a child's completion of chemotherapy, but nothing like that is scheduled for today and the exuberance of the Gazans is in marked contrast to the somber mood in the clinic.

"It's a happy day for everyone," one of the fathers explains, offering me a piece of pastry. "You get your soldier back and we get our people back. Everybody wins, everyone is happy."

I'm not sure how many of the Israelis here would agree with those sentiments, but the gesture is so genuine, their belief that today we are all winners is so palpable, that I can't help but feel moved. It must have been hard enough for the Gazans just to get through Palestinian and Israeli security that morning with their sick children, never mind carrying along the huge platters of baklava. The lives of all of these people, so different from ours, are so deeply intertwined with our own. Their children's fates are tied to our department, their homes and national aspirations affected by the same political conflict that affects our country. But more often than not, the way we see things is the exact opposite of the way they do. Our Independence Day, for example, is their Nakbah, or day of "catastrophe," during which they mourn the establishment of the State of Israel. And so I'm struck today by the effort these Palestinians have made to see this exchange not as a victory over Israel but as a shared victory, a rare instance of joint triumph deserving of mutual celebration.

The association of this land with honey goes back to the

Bible, to the book of Exodus, when God tells Moses at the burning bush that He will bring the enslaved Israelites to a land "overflowing with milk and honey." Beekeeping is a fairly big industry in Israel, and it used to be in Gaza, too. But the combined effects of cross-border shelling and Gazan urban expansion have destroyed many of the fruit trees that are necessary for the cultivation of honey. So Gazan beekeepers have in recent years moved their apiaries closer to the border with Israel, hoping that their bees, unrestrained by borders and checkpoints, will fly into Israel to gather pollen from the abundant flowers and citrus groves in the Jewish communities just over the border and then fly back to Gaza. As Israel responds to Hamas rockets with attacks of its own, the bees seem to be making the journey back and forth just fine. Oblivious to our squabbles, they do what they must to thrive. And so baklava production goes on.

As it's my last day here at Hadassah, I don't have much of an opportunity to discuss with my colleagues what they think about the Gazans' baklava gesture. Some are probably moved and heartened by it, and I'm sure others think that sending Palestinians with Israeli blood on their hands back to their homes is not something to celebrate. In any event, the children from Gaza get checked in, are assigned to rooms, and begin their chemotherapy treatments. I'll be gone by the time they're ready to leave, but the parents and staff will hopefully wrap up some of the baklava for the trip back home. It will take hours for these children to pass back through the border checkpoints, and they will be hungry.

9

The Persistence of Memory

AFTER FIVE YEARS IN THE MIDDLE EAST I am a bit shocked by the Boston weather when I arrive in December 2011. I had forgotten what New England winters could feel like, and it takes some readjusting to get used to the cold and the snow. My daily jogs along the Tel Aviv promenade, regardless of the season, are just a wistful memory now; in Boston the goal is to spend as little time outdoors as possible. Within a few weeks I figure out how to cut through the lower levels of the two shopping malls situated between my apartment and Boston Children's Hospital, zigzagging through shops and food courts in order to minimize my exposure to the cold.

I'm eager to plunge into the training program at the hospital, but I'm also not surprised to be feeling homesick for Israel—for my family and friends in Tel Aviv, and for my colleagues and patients at Hadassah. Despite being back in the country where I was born and spent most of my life, I'm in a city that's new to me and I once again feel like a new immigrant, with yet another opportunity to reinvent myself—something I find by turns exciting, scary, and a bit sad. I'm thirty-eight, and I'm still looking for home, for a place where I feel that I belong.

A MEDICAL FELLOWSHIP IS ESSENTIALLY a form of apprenticeship. It means joining a team of doctors, nurses, and social workers and learning on the job, often while bearing the brunt of the busy work. At Boston Children's Hospital it also means getting a lot of feedback and criticism of your performance. My oncology fellowship in New York had been very task-driven. For the most part you put your head down and power through the work without necessarily being overly reflective. Action was valued over introspection. Here, the opposite holds true. Every interaction, every word and gesture throughout the day, is subjected to analysis. Much of it is constructive, and I quickly feel myself developing new skills. It's like having a particularly strict trainer at the gym put you through grueling new exercises that you aren't used to, driving you through the pain until the atrophied muscles begin to gain strength. Communication skills are central to our work in palliative care, so every aspect of every interaction—with patients, with their families, and with the staff—is dissected until I am sometimes left at the end of the day feeling like the emotional equivalent of a picked-over skeleton. Why did you sit that way? Why did you make that gesture? Why did you ask this and not that? For someone like me, with more than a few years of clinical experience and already a semi-formed medical professional, the process is painful. Here I suddenly find myself not a cancer specialist managing a regional sarcoma service but a trainee in a new medical system, learning a whole new discipline.

Boston Children's has one of the oldest and most robust pediatric palliative care services in North America. It's a multidisciplinary team composed of doctors, nurse-practitioners, and social workers. As is the case with most pediatric palliative care services, and contrary to what many people assume, most of the patients they follow do not have cancer. Most are children with complex chronic illnesses, conditions defined as potentially life-limiting but where the actual course of the illness is hard to predict. These include, for example, genetic and metabolic disorders, neuromuscular disease, complex cardiac disease, and chronic lung disease. Among the most challenging situations are the ones where a child's condition is so rare and poorly understood that it's difficult even to define what the problem is beyond identifying a genetic abnormality, leaving both family and clinicians not really knowing what to expect. In these situations, it's particularly difficult to guide families in thinking about treatment decisions and medical interventions, and even just planning for life.

One of my first major adjustments in learning how to be a palliative care specialist is simply trying to figure out what my role is when I walk into a room. As an oncologist, it always felt pretty clear: I'm the doctor who is here to treat your child's cancer, albeit with no promise of success. Most oncologists' interactions with patients and families are pretty action-oriented. You see the patient, review the blood tests, look at the X-rays, MRIs, or PET scans, and move the discussion toward a treatment plan or next steps. Sometimes it's mundane (everything looks good, your blood counts are fine, see you next week for the next treatment), sometimes it's more fraught (your child's cancer has recurred, here's what that means, here are the next steps in getting treatment under way), and sometimes it's the conversation that we dread (I'm sorry, but there are no more treatments that offer a realistic hope of cure). But regardless of outcome, your role is clear: you are the doctor who treats the cancer.

The same could be said of most other specialists. The cardiologist treats ailments of the heart, the nephrologist specializes in kidney disease, and so on. But the palliative care clinician's role can be harder to define. I run into this all the time when I meet people who ask what I do. When people hear the term "palliative care," they assume it means I take care of people who are dying. This is sometimes true, but it fails to capture the majority of what we do. A palliative care team may fill any number of roles, depending on a patient's needs and the needs of her family. We might be called to help think about particularly challenging symptoms, such as complex pain management or sleep issues. Sometimes we are called to help patients and their families with difficult decision making regarding treatments or interventions. And not just the obvious ones, such as intubation and cardiac resuscitation. The discussions we are involved with encompass issues such as whether it makes sense to pursue a risky experimental therapy, have a feeding tube placed, or have a tracheostomy (an opening in the lower neck) placed to help with breathing. They are not trivial matters. These interventions may affect the way in which a patient dies, and also to what degree the family of a deceased child is left struggling with guilt and with questions about options not exercised. We will also discuss how these interventions will affect the day-to-day life of a patient—for example, how mobility may be limited for a child with a tracheostomy who is now ventilator dependent—and the patient's family. We help families think about what different pathways might look like as they unfold, and what those pathways would mean for their particular family. We provide an extra layer of support and help make sure that a child is receiving the best possible care that aligns with his family's goals and values.

It's not easy to explore hope and establish goals in a setting of prognostic uncertainty. I already knew as an oncologist that the idea of "hope" is a complex one. But for children with conditions that have wildly unpredictable trajectories and prognoses, defining what hope is becomes all the more complicated. When I started my palliative care training, I assumed that all parents hope for the same thing: that their child will get better, will walk out of the hospital healthy, and will never have to return. Asking a direct question about what parents or a patient might be hoping for seemed so obvious that it felt foolish to ask. But I learn to overcome my reservations and to probe more deeply. In doing so, or often simply by sitting silently with patients and their parents, I learn that hope—and hoping—is a far richer concept than I had suspected. I've learned to treat hope not as a noun but as a verb. Hope as a thing, as an object, can be shattered or lost. But hoping as an act doesn't ever really have to stop. And what is it that my patients and their parents are hoping for? Often I find myself talking with parents who explain that, yes, their hope once was that their child would be cured, and they would certainly love for that to happen. But if that is no longer a realistic possibility, then they are hoping for other things for their child. Things like freedom from pain, time with family, time to make memories. Whereas earlier in my career this talk of identifying new goals in the absence of cure had felt hollow, my training in palliative care began to allow me to see more fully how rich and meaningful these new goals could be. The palliative care team's task is to explore these hopes, to frame goals, and to help the patient's primary clinical teams formulate a treatment plan that will best meet these goals.

In palliative care I see families struggling with prognostic uncertainty in ways that I had not previously seen as an oncologist, or at least hadn't previously appreciated. In some ways, treating children with cancer was easy compared to this. With recurrent or progressive cancer there is an ongoing process that we may be trying to stop or to slow. But in the absence of a treatment that works, the disease process marches on, and a point is reached where death is inevitable. Now, as a palliative care doctor working with children with conditions that have such unpredictable trajectories—children who could theoretically live with their illness for years or even decades—trying to figure out how to guide them and their parents takes on a new level of difficulty. I often find at the end of an hour-long consult that I myself am struggling with the uncertainty, with no real sense of what specific recommendations to make, much to the annoyance of the child's primary care team. Our team would be called in for a consult—something along the lines of "this child and his family are falling apart, fix it"—but we would emerge with no magic button to push or pill to dispense to make it all better. I have often found that up to the very end, patients and their families are able simultaneously to understand that death is inevitable *and* to continue to hope for a cure. F. Scott Fitzgerald famously wrote that "the test of a first-rate intelligence is the ability to hold two opposing ideas in mind at the same time and still retain the ability to function." I'm learning that this is part of what it means to be human, and what keeps my patients and their families going from day to day.

OLIVER IS A FOUR-YEAR-OLD BOY who was born with holoprosencephaly, a condition in which the brain forms abnormally. The form he has is severe enough that he shows very little outward function—mostly just rolling his eyes, smacking his lips, and fairly constant writhing movements of his limbs, all of which are involuntary. When I meet him for the first time during an admission for treatment of pneumonia, I can see that he doesn't interact with or respond to the world around him at all. He doesn't make eye contact, doesn't respond to any stimuli, and exhibits no purposeful movements. His mother, a single parent, has built her entire life around his needs, and from hearing her story it's clear that most of her days must revolve around caring for him. At that first meeting I ask her, as my palliative care mentors have been training me to do, what Oliver is like as child: what are his likes and dislikes, what is a good day for him and what is a bad day? I feel foolish asking all this, since it's evident that he is without any real cognition. So I am taken aback when his mother launches into a long description of what a sweet child he is, how most days he is very happy, how he loves classic rock music and being outside on sunny days. Anticipating my next question, she explains that Oliver gives her yes-or-no answers to her questions by looking either to the left or to the right. But as I watch him writhing on the bed, his eyes rolling around aimlessly, my heart goes out to this woman; there is no way Oliver has the capacity to think, let alone convey his thoughts. It's beautiful to see how much Oliver's mom loves and cares for her child, but also a bit sad that she's living with such delusions.

Over the course of my time at Boston Children's, Oliver is admitted to the hospital with some regularity, and I get to know him and his mother better. And with time I become more attuned to nuances I might never have paid attention to. Sitting in Oliver's room while I chat with his mother, at a certain point I believe I can *almost* see for myself when he is moving his eyes in response to her questions. I'm never really sure; it might simply be my imagination and the result of my spending so much (too much?) time in their room. But I also realize that it doesn't really matter whether Oliver is actually communicating with his mother through purposeful eye movements or she's just imagining it. What matters is how she perceives him as a little boy and how she has constructed a world for them together.

Pediatric palliative care is about learning to see a child and his family through different eyes, to become attuned to language and environment in new ways. Our team's conversations with families are wide-ranging and involve open-ended questions, such as "What sort of person is your child?" or "What are you hoping for and what are you most worried about?" The objective is, over the course of time, to get a sense of what the goals of the child and family are, and what is important to them. Only then can we make suggestions about which clinical decisions might be most appropriate for a particular child and his family. I think back to the patients I had cared for as an oncologist who had been removed from treatment protocols because of the inexorable progression of their disease. I am able to articulate now what I only intuited back then, that no matter how scary it is not to have a map, in being "lost" there is also opportunity. Of course, no one wants to end up in a situation where there is no established treatment protocol, but with the right guide that journey can still be meaningful. To paraphrase Herman Melville, the truest places never are down on a map. And it's our job to go to those truest places with our patients.

Oliver develops aspiration pneumonia with increasing frequency. After multiple intensive-care admissions and near intubations, the primary team begins to press his mother to consider having a tracheostomy placed. But they call us in frustration when she tells them repeatedly that Oliver has told her that he doesn't want a tracheostomy. In our team's conversations with her, she tells us that Oliver is worried that having a tracheostomy will be uncomfortable and will not really add to his quality of life as he sees it. He worries that the next step will be to attach the tracheostomy to a ventilator and that this will be the start of a slippery slope that will end with his being completely technology-dependent, being kept alive in the intensive care unit but unable to do anything. The primary care team becomes even more unsettled when we report this discussion back to them. They argue that the fact that Oliver's mother has, to their minds, imagined the entire dialogue with her son simply calls her sanity further into question and also raises serious ethical questions. But with time we are able to help guide them through several more conversations with her. We emphasize that whether or not these conversations between Oliver and his mom are happening in the way we conceive of normal dialogue is irrelevant; what's important is that this is her perception of what her son wants and is therefore a reflection of her values and beliefs. If we are all wrong and, no matter how impossible it seems, Oliver is in fact communicating with her, she has made clear she wants to honor his wishes. And if she is simply reporting her own values and wishes refracted through how she sees Oliver, then that is also a set of values and goals that we as a medical team need to help support.

Palliative care means seeing engagement with a patient and her family as more of a process than the achievement of a specific, immediate solution. Being comfortable with not coming up with concrete answers becomes a new skill set in my clinical toolbox. I learn to get to the end of a consultation and conclude by saying, "Well, this is the start of an ongoing conversation. To be continued." There are, of course, times when families themselves seem a bit confused by this, accustomed more to traditional, focused, plan-driven clinical interactions. Some families respond politely at the end of the hour with slightly confused looks. "Yes," they repeat, somewhat bewildered, "to be continued," clearly wondering what they have just spent an hour of their valuable time doing with our team. Some, unsure of what to do with that lack of clarity, fill in the blank space themselves, with whatever they feel is a results-oriented outcome. "So, uh, you'll get us that wheelchair/flight to Arizona/trip to Disney World/experimental drug?" they ask, having decided that our team is some version of social worker, pharmacy, or charity.

CHARLIE IS AN EIGHTEEN-YEAR-OLD with cystic fibrosis, a condition in which patients have trouble clearing secretions from their lungs, leading to recurrent infections and progressively worsening pulmonary function. Though with good care patients may live for decades, much of their daily existence depends on complex regimens of medications and physical therapy to stave off any worsening of their condition. For a patient with cystic fibrosis, something as minor as a bad cold can quickly spin out of control and lead to significant unanticipated deterioration. Charlie was diagnosed with the disease when he was three years old; by now he has pretty poor lung function and is becoming progressively dependent on oxygen, which he can administer himself at home via portable oxygen tanks. Because of his diminished lung function, Charlie is tired most of the time and feels increasingly limited in what he can do with his friends. When he does go out, he has to tote along a small oxygen tank, which he finds both cumbersome and embarrassing. Though the smaller tank allows for greater portability, it also holds less oxygen, so Charlie has to pay constant attention to how much reserve is left and make sure to get home before it runs out. When I first meet him, Charlie has just been admitted with a viral infection, and the pulmonary team asks us to get involved to help manage his increasing sense of breathlessness. They also ask us to begin exploring goals of care with him and his family so that we would be better able to guide them should a tracheostomy or a lung transplant eventually become an option that needs to be explored. Charlie's parents, immigrants from Egypt, welcome our team's presence, but they are very protective of their son and ask at first that we not meet alone with him. The outdated stereotype of the palliative care team as the "death squad" is hard to break; many families fear that our involvement is a sign that death is approaching or that all we want to talk about is end-of-life issues. We honor Charlie's parents' request, even though at age eighteen he is legally an adult and able to make his own decisions, hoping that with time we will be able to gain their trust and develop a relationship with them. The first few meetings are a bit stilted, as my colleagues and I try to get a feel for who this family is and what is important to them, all the while carefully avoiding the obvious fact that Charlie is wearing a special face mask forcing oxygen under pressure up through his nostrils and into his lungs as he tries to talk to us between breaths.

At the end of our third visit, as we get up to leave the room, I ask Charlie whether there is anything we can do for him, anything we can bring him.

"Well," he said, "I have to be honest with you. You guys seem really nice and all, but I'm still not really sure what you're doing here."

We all laugh. I get it. In honoring his parents' request not to address directly the issue of Charlie's cystic fibrosis, we are still looking for some other role during our meetings, some other way to get "buy in" with this family.

"You're right," I say, "sometimes it takes a while not just for patients but for us as well to figure out where we fit in. We'll keep stopping by, and with time we'll see if there's anything we can do to help."

Slowly, over the course of weeks, our team develops a relationship with Charlie. We win some good faith by suggesting a medication that helps with his feeling of breathlessness. His parents begin to allow us to spend time alone with him. As they become less suspicious of us, they even start offering us sweets or tea with each visit. I feel a twinge of homesickness for Israel as I sip mint tea and nibble sesame cookies, dredging up some of my limited Arabic while we chat.

But despite our developing relationship with Charlie and his family, there is always a sense that we are being held at arm's length, that they are still unwilling to allow us into their lives at anything but a superficial level. Then one day I notice a collection of Eastern Orthodox religious icons that Charlie has assembled on the windowsill. One of the tricks I learn in palliative care training is to be aware of cues in a patient's room that might provide an insight into who he is and what's important to him. With my interest in spirituality, I often find myself looking for hints such as a rosary pinned to a pillow or a prayer taped to the wall. When I ask about the icons, Charlie lights up. He launches into an animated lecture on who each of the saints is and what each of them means to him. I share my own background in religious studies. The icons and spirituality turn into the basis for an ongoing discussion, and before I know it these discussions have evolved to encompass his illness as well. Soon we've established enough trust that we're having conversations I never thought we'd get to.

Though the idea had initially been for our team to help optimize Charlie's quality of life outside the hospital, the admission hasn't gone as planned. Every time a potential discharge date approaches, another complication surfaces, either a fever or a cold. It's becoming apparent that Charlie might never leave the hospital, at least not without a major intervention such as the placement of a tracheostomy. In the end, events move more quickly than anyone had anticipated. Complications snowball and Charlie's condition worsens precipitously. During what turns out to be his final two weeks of life, our team has become a major source of support for Charlie and his family. We've gone from relatively short and somewhat awkward visits to spending huge chunks of our day in his room. We no longer have to strategize about how to get into discussions about the big issues; by this point in our relationship they seek our input. When it comes time to make decisions about whether to limit attempts at resuscitation, our team is at Charlie's bedside providing guidance, right up until the moment when his heart stops. One morning, as I'm out for an early jog, the sun not even up yet, my pager goes off, warning me that the end seems near. I jog the rest of the way to the hospital and throw on a pair of scrubs, joining my colleagues outside Charlie's room. The room, dark except for a dim bedside lamp throwing a halo of light onto Charlie's pale face, is crowded with family. I think of all the times I had witnessed similar moments at Hadassah. The sheets are drawn up to Charlie's chin, and it's clear that he is no longer breathing. His mother looks up from the bedside and, seeing us through the open door, calls us in, saying, "Come. Come say goodbye to your friend."

Our friend. It's one of the most memorable moments of my training. How remarkable, to go in just a few months from not being sure what our role is to being regarded as friends who were there for a young man and his family as his life ebbed away.

. . .

DURING MY ONCOLOGY FELLOWSHIP I had developed an interest in photography. I loved the blend of science and art, and the few hours a week I could arrange for darkroom time provided a welcome respite from the stress of work. I could close myself away in, literally, a dark room, which was completely silent except for the not unpleasant sound of water dripping into the rinsing basin. Warm, vinegary clouds of chemicals would waft agreeably through my head. My only focus was the pool of light in front of me, my only concern the hypnotic process of exposing and printing images in the dark. I would step out of the darkroom to evaluate each print, debating where to crop, where to enlarge, where to burn in more deeply. Photos that I had snapped carelessly (or poorly), which on first inspection seemed blurry or uninteresting, could often be mined for luscious detail, resulting in a powerful and unexpected image.

In *On Photography* and *Regarding the Pain of Others,* Susan Sontag famously writes about the interaction between viewer and subject when a person looks at a photograph of someone who is suffering or dying. She explains how the interaction differs when the subject is making eye contact with the camera and when he isn't. This assertion challenges me to think about how I observe my patients. Am I the dispassionate clinician, observing a patient solely to determine the best course of medical intervention? Or am I also engaging with the patient I'm looking at, and in the process trying to imagine what she is feeling and thinking? Is it possible to do both? Isn't it necessary to do both? These lessons from photography come to mind as I develop my skills in palliative care. So much of what we do in palliative care depends on careful observation: on noticing the details, whether it's the icons on the windowsill, the glances between worried parents, or the pregnant silence before a question is asked. These are the sorts of things that are easily missed. Worse, they are the sorts of things that are easily dismissed and ignored. But observing them, exploring them, those little hints and details are what allow us to develop the smallest openings into the most meaningful spaces. I had glimpsed this before, but Boston is where I learn to cultivate this as a skill.

There is, however, a downside to assuming the role of observer. If I'm not actively contributing to patient care, I run the risk of turning into a voyeur. "Perhaps the only people with the right to look at images of suffering of this extreme order," Sontag writes, "are those who could do something to alleviate it ... or those who could learn from it. The rest of us are voyeurs, whether or not we mean to be." Which is why it's important to acknowledge that what our palliative care team does is ultimately goal-oriented, the goal being to extract useful information ("actionable intelligence," to use the military term) from every interaction with a patient and/or her family. What I try to learn during this fellowship is how to find the balance between observation and action, between being and doing, silence and speech.

IN NOVEMBER 2012, midway through my fellowship, another round of violence breaks out between Israel and the Hamas fighters in Gaza. Though I feel a tug of guilt at not being there, it's not enough to make me abandon my program and get on a plane to Tel Aviv. I go about my work and follow the news of the increasing tensions, but I assume that this latest crisis will, like most flare-ups, quickly dissipate. Then one morning as I'm making rounds in the hospital my mother in Tel Aviv calls my cellphone. It takes only a few seconds for me to realize that the strange background noise I'm hearing is an air-raid siren, and that it's going off not in a town close to the Gaza border but in my old neighborhood of Neve Tzedek, where my parents and my brother and his family now live.

"Is that an air-raid siren?" I ask, rather stupidly, not wanting to believe what I'm hearing.

Before she can answer there is a loud explosion on her end of the phone. A Hamas rocket has hit something nearby, and my mother, terrified, just keeps saying, "Oh, shit. Oh, shit." But my parents' building appears to be okay. My mother calms down enough to get my father to come in from the porch, where he is trying to see if he can tell where the rocket landed, and go with her to their designated shelter until the sirens stop.

I spend the next few days agonizing over whether I should go back to Israel. My reserve unit has not been activated and I'm still on leave from Hadassah, so I'm not sure what I would do there if I did go back. Disrupting my fellowship just to sit at home with my family would serve no purpose. So I wait, trying to focus on my work but feeling guilty about not being in Israel while the country is under attack. If my reserve unit is called up I will definitely join them, and I decide that even if it isn't activated but the war expands, I will return. But a cease-fire is announced relatively quickly, and the tense calm punctuated by brief acts of violence that passes for peace resumes.

It's around this time that our pediatric palliative care team becomes involved in the care of Mark, a teenage boy with an incurable brain tumor. It's a rare type of tumor, and because of its unique location Mark's only symptoms so far are headaches and an inability to create new memories. Otherwise, he appears to be just fine, and if you met him in passing you would never know that he harbors a ticking time bomb in his head. Our team's interactions with Mark are surreal. At every visit we introduce ourselves, ask one or two questions to see how he is feeling, and then engage him in conversation. After a few minutes there is a brief pause, and we can almost hear the click of a reset button in Mark's head as he stares off into space, his eyes losing focus, and then suddenly he looks back at us and says, "Hi, who are you?"

Our team is asked to help Mark with his headaches and to help guide him and his family through the difficult decisions facing them. There are immediate interventions to consider— surgery, radiation, chemotherapy—and, eventually, advance care

planning and thinking about what the end might look like. But
this situation seems particularly unique and poignant. Normally
we explore goals and values by exploring *who* a person is, what
imparts meaning to a given family when thinking about how
life may unfold. But how do we establish goals and values when
there is nothing but the present moment? How do we create
meaning or make plans if our patient has no memories, no recognition of context? How do we provide guidance when every
visit is just a repeat of the previous one? Mark's family settles
into a painful pattern, simply living day by day, hour by hour,
finding meaning and value in each interaction, even if it seems
to be the same thing over and over. The changes are impercep-
tible at first, but as the weeks pass Mark begins to slow down,
become more confused, then sleepy, until he finally slips away.

I DO NOT—THANK GOD—HAVE A FATAL brain tumor,
but I, too, seem to be unable to chart a future course of action
for myself. For much of my time in Boston I date a woman who,
though lovely, is a Catholic Republican and pretty much my
opposite, and it's not clear where that is heading. At one point
in the middle of the fellowship I grow so unsure of myself that
I actually interview at the management consulting firm McKin-
sey & Company, thinking that perhaps I should change careers
altogether. How do I create a meaningful life and make decisions
about how to live it if I seem to be fixated on erasing the person
I used be? How do I plan for my own life if I am unable to put
down roots anywhere and instead spend my time hopping from
place to place, constantly re-creating myself? My experience in
Boston has certainly helped me develop as a clinician, but as far
as developing a better sense of self, not so much.

I'm in a taxi one Friday morning on the way to work when
my five-year-old nephew and two-year-old niece call me on the
phone from Tel Aviv. My nephew's got a splinter in his finger,

and he insists that his mother call me so that, via Skype, he can show me his finger and consult with me on his condition. (He has by this time figured out that I'm a pediatrician, though he remains blissfully ignorant of my subspecialties.) After I offer him some reassurance, the three of us start joking around, the kids updating me on what's new in their lives that week. When their mother calls out that it's time to get off the phone, they begin shouting over each other, telling me that they love me and miss me, and wishing me a Shabbat shalom.

The driver looks at me in the rearview mirror as I put my phone away.

"Man," he says, "what are you doing here? It sounds to me like they need you there!"

Back at home that night I flip through the pictures of Israel on my computer. I think about how we look at images, how we seek that balance between observation and action. Professionally, I want to be able to do both, and my heart tells me to return to Israel with my newly acquired skills, to bring this new discipline of pediatric palliative care to the place I still very much want to call home.

I remember what it was that I was searching for when I first moved to Israel. I recall the people I left behind there, the goals that I'd sought to achieve, the meaning I had hoped my life would have. Starting a formal pediatric palliative care service at Hadassah, the first of its kind in Israel, will give me a new sense of focus. I decide that I'm going to give this one more shot, and I start planning.

While I'm in Boston I have become aware that Hadassah is undergoing a period of financial hardship. There are occasional stories in the Israeli newspapers hinting at instability, and I hear from colleagues that a consulting firm has been hired to help with restructuring. The story going around is that Hadassah, not the most financially robust institution in the Israeli health-care system to begin with, has lost a fortune in Bernard Madoff's investment scandal. That loss, combined with the cost of a massive new building that is under construction, is straining the financial underpinnings of the hospital. But, I reason to myself, this is *Hadassah,* which is, after all, synonymous with Israeli pride and biomedical innovation. Hadassah, the Women's Zionist Organization of America, the American fundraising powerhouse that had been the driving force behind the development of the hospital back in the 1930s, has always backed the place financially; surely it would continue to do so forever.

Aware of Hadassah's situation but armed with a sense of mission, I fly to Israel in early 2013, as my fellowship draws to a close, to see my family and to meet with the managing director of the hospital. We'd had a cordial relationship in the past—a former high-ranking officer in the Medical Corps, he had helped me navigate the system when I was first drafted—and he welcomes me into his office, even though I know he must be distracted by the presence of people from the consulting firm who are just beginning their on-site analysis.

Moving quickly past pleasantries, I hand him a folder with my business plan and proposed budget, pitching my vision for the development of a pediatric palliative care service at Hadassah. This would be, to the best of my knowledge, the first dedicated pediatric palliative care service in the Middle East, and it would be headed by the only fellowship-trained and board-eligible pediatric palliative care physician in Israel.

"I love the idea," he says, setting the papers aside. "But how many beds do you want?"

For a hospital administrator, beds and all that go with them—space, equipment, personnel—are the main currency in operational planning. Beds mean everything. They cost money and, depending on how they are utilized, they can also make money. And of course it's easier to think in terms of beds than in terms of human lives or sick children.

"None," I say. "I just need salaries for clinicians and a small additional amount for things like education and materials. Most of what we'll be doing as a consult service will be engaging in conversations and making recommendations for families and primary care teams."

His eyes light up, and I can practically hear his internal calculator kicking into high gear. I feel the same way that I do when shopping for trinkets in the market in Jerusalem's Old City, when both the shopkeeper and I have tipped our hands just enough to know that we're both interested in making the sale, and the real bargaining is about to start.

"You know," he says slowly, "this is not a great time for Hadassah. We're just starting to look at restructuring, and we're really looking for ways to cut costs, not to fund new initiatives."

"Well," I reply, fully prepared for this response, "palliative care may not seem like a big moneymaker, but there is plenty of evidence that it's a cost avoider, which may sound less sexy but still would save the hospital money, bottom line. Plus, I've been meeting with potential donors in the United States, and I think there may be real interest in supporting this. I mean, what cause could be more meaningful than helping Arab and Jewish kids facing life-threatening illness under one roof? And having the first palliative care service in Israel certainly wouldn't hurt Hadassah's image, especially if the place is going through a rough patch right now."

"Donors?" he says, suddenly alarmed by what is obviously a very loaded term. "You'll have to be very careful. You absolutely cannot touch any existing Hadassah donors. We're working hard to direct money to existing deficits, like paying for the completion of the new tower. But if you have other connections. . . . If you can bring in this money—and I have full faith that you can—I don't see any reason why this can't happen."

I try not to look too excited as I smile and assure him that I will keep away from current Hadassah donors in my fundraising. We shake hands, both of us very pleased by the outcome of our negotiation, and I leave, pretty happy with myself. On the drive back to Tel Aviv I realize that I have just made my second serious commitment to the Hadassah Medical Center, but with a more sharply defined goal and sense of purpose, I feel that this time I have a better chance of success. It's only later in the day, as I recount the conversation to my family, that it occurs to me that the great deal I have just negotiated is essentially a handshake that authorizes me to go ahead and bring Hadassah a lot of money without any firm commitment from them. I shake off the feeling that I have not crossed all the *t*'s and dotted all the *i*'s, that perhaps I should have gotten some of this in writing. I tell myself that this must be how it's done at upper-management levels, that money talks, and that if I raise the necessary amount I'll have my program and will be able to do everything I've planned.

When I return to Boston I get down to the task of fundraising. I'd taught myself as much as possible about business planning and program development from books and from talking to colleagues in other hospitals in North America about how they had developed their own services. I begin networking my way through potential donors, shamelessly pitching the project at every opportunity. I also develop a small group of allies in New York and Boston, people who introduce me to potential donors, give me fundraising advice, and even organize a few speaking events where I promote the cause. By August I have enough potential major donors expressing serious interest that I feel I can go back to Jerusalem and start laying the groundwork for the new service. I return to Hadassah in September, and with part of my time officially allocated to developing a program for pediatric palliative care, I'm more convinced than ever of my purpose.

10

Little Wins

A S EXCITED AS I AM ABOUT starting to build the new
program at Hadassah, I'm also fully aware that successfully
implementing it is going to be an uphill battle. Had I decided to
remain in the United States, I would likely have been able to land
a comfortable job in an established pediatric palliative care program. Here in Israel I will be creating a new subspecialty almost
from scratch, and in a culture that initially is probably not going
to be all that receptive. But I'm convinced in my heart that with
this new program I will be able to effect positive change here in a
way that I never would be able to in America, and I'm possessed
by an almost Divine certainty that I am fulfilling my destiny.

But beyond my ideas for fundraising, I don't really have a
plan in place for how to create my program. I have a rough business plan, a number of donor contacts, and a vague sense of
how I imagine the pediatric palliative care service rolling out. I
even decide to live in Jerusalem, away from friends and family
in Tel Aviv, so that I will be more easily available in off-hours

once the program gets started. I had spent a good chunk of my time at Boston Children's trying to dissect their very successful program, to figure out exactly how it had evolved, how it now functioned, and how it might be successfully exported to Jerusalem. The business and management literature I'd read gave me pointers on how to grow a team, how to start something new from scratch, how to sell an idea. In Israel, palliative care is still very much seen as just hospice and end-of-life care, which of course is not the message I want to convey. When I excitedly describe to colleagues at Hadassah what I had learned in Boston and what I hope to set up here, they say things like, "Great, now we'll have you to help us when it's time to transition our end-of-life kids to palliative care." I patiently explain to them that pediatric palliative care is actually about providing a broad spectrum of support for children and their families, regardless of the patient's prognosis. That it deals with exploring all sorts of goals of care and making sure that the best possible care in line with a family's values is being delivered. I tell them that it's not about "transitioning" but about concurrently providing that extra layer of support, even while a patient is being given disease-directed therapy and the family is hoping for a cure. That's when they all get the same pained expression.

"So you basically just talk?" they say, managing to sound simultaneously confused and disdainful. "That's what you learned? That's so American."

The management at Hadassah, desperately trying to stave off the looming financial crisis, can offer me nothing more than their own peculiar form of moral support.

"Keep working on the donors," they tell me. "*Yih'yeh b'seder,* it'll be fine. Just bring us the money."

To be fair, there are individuals at Hadassah who are very receptive and attuned to the nuances of pediatric palliative care, especially within my own Department of Pediatric Hematology-Oncology, and they are a strong source of support for me. In fact, I'm convinced that my relationships with them, as well as the unique relationships we clinicians have with our patients in this particularly fraught part of the world, have served as the catalyst for my decision to redirect my career in this way. There's something so intensely up close and personal about life here in Israel—in one's professional life as well as in one's personal life—that forces you as a clinician to see your patients and their families in a way that is very different from what I have experienced in the United States.

There are some unexpected allies in other departments as well. One is a pediatric rheumatologist who specializes in autoimmune and joint diseases. I introduce myself to her shortly after returning from Boston, seeking help for myself. After experiencing years of intermittent back pain, I had been diagnosed in Boston with a form of arthritis for which I was started on an anti-inflammatory medication. Faced with muddling through the Israeli healthcare system to get approval for the same medication I had already been successfully taking in America, I've become enough of a local to look for a path of lesser resistance. And so I rely on *protektzia,* or connections, appealing directly to the rheumatologist to do me a favor and just write me a prescription.

We chat for a while, and she is kind enough to help me out. A few weeks later, she calls me looking for a favor in return. She has been caring for Sami, an eight-year-old Palestinian boy from a village near Bethlehem who has been suffering for years from a poorly defined chronic autoimmune disease. She's tried multiple treatment regimens over the years, but each new drug either worked for only a limited time or failed outright. She is out of options, she says, except for one or two highly experimental and potentially dangerous medications. In the meantime, Sami is suffering terribly, and his symptoms are poorly controlled. Could I come by and see if I have any thoughts? Thrilled by this outreach from an unexpected direction, as well as by the fact that this is not a strict end-of-life consultation, I eagerly agree.

I'm determined to put my most professional foot forward. "Little wins" are what all of the management books I've been reading recommend; focus on small victories, and eventually they will add up to create a thriving business (or, in my case, a thriving new service). I look forward to demonstrating symptom management skills, elucidating the goals of care, and helping with decision making. As I wait for the elevator I review in my head the elements of a good initial consult, feeling like an athlete before a big game. I will sit quietly with the family, explain my role, and take as much time as necessary to get to know who they are, who Sami is, and what is most important to them. Then, having established a meaningful rapport with the family, I will package what I have learned into a well-written report for my colleagues that will help guide the primary care team and the family through future decisions regarding Sami's course of treatment. I'm all set to dazzle them, Boston-style.

There is an old military saying that no battle plan survives first contact with the enemy. The elevator door opens and it's like hitting the beach on D-day. The clinic is packed and in utter chaos, with adults yelling, kids crying, and no discernible sense of order or organization. When I finally locate the rheumatologist, she is with Sami and his parents, all of them crammed into a tiny room that contains a small desk, three chairs, and an examination table, all more or less on top of one another. The room is otherwise bare: no decorations, no medical diagrams, not even a calendar. Just four walls with blistered and peeling paint. The paper-thin door barely muffles the racket from the waiting area. Also in the room is a man acting as an Arabic interpreter. I can't tell if he is a family member or a random passerby who has been pressed into service, and when I ask, all I get by way of response is "he's a relative," which could still mean just about anything and is conveyed in a tone that tells me not to ask for details.

Sami is curled up on his side in a fetal position on the exam table. When I go to put a hand on him to say hello, I realize that he is curled up not because that is how he is most comfortable but because his spine and limbs are so deformed from years of inflammation that he is now stuck in this position. Between the noise outside, the cramped space, the parents' obvious fatigue, and the general feeling of distress in the room generated by the presence of a suffering child, my plans for a model consult evaporate. There is no way I can go through the entire initial consult as I had planned. Instead, I focus on evaluating Sami's symptoms. It doesn't take long to ascertain that he is in tremendous, constant pain and that he is barely getting even the simplest over-the-counter pain medicines. He hasn't slept a full night in months, and he is severely malnourished, both because he has no appetite due to the pain and because he can't move his arms enough to feed himself or his neck enough to allow anyone else to adequately feed him. His parents, red-eyed and haggard, are clearly exhausted. When I ask about their home life, his mother confesses that she hasn't had much sleep, either, because every night she sits in bed with Sami, trying her best to hold him in a comfortable position.

Focusing on Sami's pain, I suggest that we try giving him methadone, an inexpensive and very effective pain medicine, albeit one that requires close follow-up to make sure it's being properly adjusted as needed. Even a suggestion as simple as this will take a bit of explanation and some modest legwork, as methadone cannot be reliably obtained in the West Bank. We get a supply from the hospital pharmacy and, after I explain its use to my colleague and to Sami's parents, we send them home with a plan for the rheumatologist to follow up by phone in a few days. The full consult will have to wait until he is feeling better.

Four days later I receive a message from the rheumatologist: Sami has slept straight through the night for the first time in months. She is beside herself with relief, and we agree to set up an appointment for the following week so that I can do a better evaluation of Sami and continue to get to know the family.

At the next visit Sami seems to be feeling better, though he is still severely limited by his limb contractures and still badly, even dangerously, malnourished. With some pleading we receive permission from the PA Health Ministry to admit him to the hospital for nutritional support and placement of a feeding tube. The process of getting permission is not simple. Though in my eyes nutritional support pretty clearly constitutes a lifesaving intervention in this case, explaining that to some bureaucrat in the PA proves to be far more difficult than explaining why chemotherapy is necessary for a child with cancer.

As often happens with children who have a complex chronic illness, Sami's hospital stay quickly becomes more complicated than planned. He develops a number of ancillary problems, including increasing systemic inflammation and trouble breathing, which places his life in real, immediate danger. Having barely begun to get to know this family, I'm asked to help establish whether Sami should be intubated and put on a ventilator if he becomes sicker, or if limiting such interventions is in line with the family's values and goals, given that intubation would likely not save him and will simply prolong his dying process.

His father comes to the hospital infrequently, afraid of losing his job if he is absent too often, so most of my interactions are with Sami's mother. In the course of talking everything through with me, she expresses her feeling that Sami's life as it currently stands involves enormous suffering. Though she still wants to pursue any possible curative interventions, including the experimental options under consideration, she also feels that if an acute, life-threatening event occurs, she would not want any heroic attempts at resuscitation.

The degree of distress that this decision causes among some of the staff catches me by surprise. I convey Sami's mother's wishes to the inpatient team managing his care and help the residents enter a "do not resuscitate" (DNR) order in Sami's chart. I'm feeling pretty good about myself, having clarified goals and put down clear parameters for the staff in case anything cata-strophic were to happen. But before I can leave for the day I am confronted by another physician whom I barely know. He screams at me, asking how I could dare discuss limitations of interventions with a parent when there are still drugs, albeit experimental, that have not been tried. Other staff members express confusion: has the patient been formally "transitioned" to palliative care or not? Though some of the clinicians, like my screaming colleague, are difficult to convince, most of the staff are receptive to my attempts to explain to them the nuances of Sami's care, and they embrace this "new" concept of being able simultaneously to explore limiting some types of interventions while still hoping for benefit from others that have yet to be tried.

In the end, one of the experimental drugs helps and Sami improves enough to be released from the hospital. With some additional pleading we are able to get permission from the PA to admit him to an Israeli rehabilitation facility, where he continues to gain weight and regain some use of his arms and legs. Sami's underlying illness will likely flare up again at some point, but for the time being he is well on his way to dramatically improved health.

With this initial experience in pediatric palliative care at Hadassah, I can already feel how much I've changed through my exposure to pediatric palliative care in Boston. There was a time when I also would have looked at the issues of treatment and limitations of intervention in more black-and-white, either/or terms. Years earlier, as a trainee beginning an overnight shift, when faced with the prospect of a seriously ill child potentially becoming less stable, I would anxiously ask if a DNR order had been obtained. Worse yet, I would feel relieved if the answer was yes, as though I was therefore absolved of having to go into that room, of having to engage with the family at all. Now I see things in a much less binary way. Patient care is not an either/

or construct, cure-driven or comfort-driven. Decisions and goals can be, and usually are, much more nuanced. Critically ill children, just like critically ill grown-ups, have ever-changing hopes, fears, and goals. And our approach to the treatment of children naturally occurs within the context of the family unit, with both the patient and her parents bringing their own values and concerns to the table, so that a complex but complete picture can be formed and decisions made accordingly. But my experience with the rest of the staff during Sami's treatment also makes clear how much work I still have to do to bridge the culture gap here.

WHEN FOURTEEN-YEAR-OLD FARHAN is wheeled into our clinic by his father for the first time, his face is heartbreakingly grotesque. A huge tumor, originating somewhere on the internal surface of his skull between his right eye and upper jaw, has distorted the entire right side of his face, twisting it into a mess of lumps and ridges. The tissue around his right eye is swollen to several times its normal size so that it protrudes out of his face, distended and meaty, with an amphibian-looking lid pulled tightly over it. His mouth has been forced open by the tumor, which protrudes out past his teeth as a hard, white mass that I'd at first mistaken for a wad of gauze. His head lolls to one side as he moans, conscious but unable to communicate.

The tumor, which turns out to be an osteosarcoma, has grown rapidly in just a few weeks. What had started as a toothache and suspected infection has become this deforming, life-threatening mass, as his parents frantically tried to find a doctor who could help, first within the PA healthcare system and finally, after it was apparent that this was likely cancer, at Hadassah.

Farhan is quickly shuttled from the waiting area to an exam room, where he remains for the rest of the day's visit, in large part for the sake of the rest of the patients in the clinic. Even in pediatric oncology, where staff and families alike are accustomed to seeing things that would elicit stares or gasps on the street, Farhan's appearance would shock the most seasoned clinician.

It takes several days for the scans to be completed and the biopsy results to be confirmed. In the meantime, Farhan is admitted to the ward and we focus on pain and symptom management. In many respects I am filling the role of both oncologist and palliative care clinician at the same time. With the help of an Arabic interpreter we explain to him at each step what we are doing and, eventually, what chemotherapy will be like. He's far too ill to be responsive, but we go through the motions and hope that he hears us. As the chemotherapy kicks in, over the course of several weeks, the tumor slowly begins to shrink. One day while examining him I realize that he can actually close his mouth and is starting to be able to open his right eye, which is by now slightly less swollen. With the shrinking of the tumor, we begin to see an improvement in Farhan's behavior. His personality begins to emerge, and we discover that he is a terrific kid. I spend hours talking with him and his family through an interpreter, explaining our plans for continued treatment. I try my best to cultivate a cautious optimism, all the while knowing that the outcome is far from certain and that the hardest parts of treatment still lie ahead. Farhan's father often ends our visits by promising that, at the end of therapy, they will invite me to their village and slaughter a sheep in honor of the occasion. I don't think they realize how difficult it would be for me to get to their village, which is deep in the West Bank. I briefly fantasize about making such a visit, even though I know, having spent some of my time in the army in the adjacent hills, that their village is not a place I could easily or safely go to.

We slowly gain control over the tumor and return Farhan to some semblance of a life. Eventually, we are able to discharge him and continue his treatment on an outpatient basis. Several months into his chemotherapy, I am joined on rounds one day by a visiting American medical student. Walking through the ward, I point out different patients, reeling off a basic outline of each child's story and treatment. Farhan has been admitted for his latest round of chemotherapy, and I wave to him as I pause outside his open door. He sits up, the cherry-red medication running into his body from the IV bag hanging at his bedside, and he smiles and waves back. Farhan's face is still misshapen from the tumor, and though his appearance has dramatically improved, I can see that the medical student is staring.

"This is one of my favorite patients," I tell the student, even though we're really not supposed to think of our patients in those terms. I launch into a brief recounting of how he had arrived at our clinic, and how well he is responding to therapy.

"So," I conclude, "we're happy so far, but of course there's still a long road ahead, with surgery and more treatments." I wave goodbye to Farhan before moving on.

"You know," Farhan suddenly says, "I speak English."

I almost faint. "You what?" I say, staring at him.

"Yes," he says, smiling. "I speak English."

"Why haven't you ever told me?" I exclaim. "I'm embarrassed! How have you let me talk to you all these months through an interpreter without telling me you speak English?"

"You never asked," he says matter-of-factly.

He's right, of course. I smile and walk over to take his hand. There's no end to the surprises, good and bad, one encounters in practicing medicine.

After months of chemotherapy, major surgery, and a complicated recovery, we get to a point where scans show no evidence of disease in Farhan's body. But the surgery is disfiguring, almost as much as the tumor itself had been. With the underlying tumor removed and the surrounding fat and muscle stripped away, the right side of his face is now sunken and scarred, and deep depressions replace the jagged masses that had protruded months before. Even though we all feel that Farhan's appearance has been greatly improved, this is partly because we have all become used to it. And in getting to know him, we've all been able to see beyond his appearance. His face has a peculiarly cubist appearance, all flattened planes and perspectives, like something drawn by Picasso. I am increasingly aware of how my palliative care training has affected my practice as an oncologist. I spend more time than I previously might have exploring with Farhan and his family what they have made of all this, and what they are hoping for. Although I am trying to remain optimistic, I know he is at a very high risk for a recurrence. And so slowly, gently, I also begin to explore with them what sorts of things we should be thinking about if everything doesn't go as planned, what would be most important to them. All of our imaging studies, CT scans, MRIs, pathology reports, and molecular studies give us one kind of picture of our patients. We scour them, trying to decipher not only what type of tumor the patient has but also how it will respond and what it will do. Though our imaging studies may reveal a great deal of information, they are just snapshots of a moment, perhaps offering suggestions about a tumor's nature and likely progression but nothing that definitively tells us how the life of this particular patient with this particular disease will play out. For insight into that, I need to get to know my patients in a different way. I need to try to figure out who they are, what their goals are, and what I can do to help them achieve these goals. In Farhan's case, this has meant a risky and disfiguring treatment in order to obtain the best chance for disease-free survival.

The clinicians who have been taking care of Farhan are not the only ones who have become deeply affected by their involvement with this special young man. The volunteers who are fulfilling their National Service requirement in our department become attached to Farhan in a way that I have never seen them do with any other Arab child. In fact, when it comes time for the annual weeklong trip to Europe that their sponsoring organization runs, to their great credit they jump through hoops to arrange for Farhan to travel with them.

Taking any sort of trip with children who are being treated

for cancer can be incredibly complicated. Even a day trip to a local park can require enormous preparation and logistical support. Not only do you need to have easy access to a doctor or a nurse, you also need to make sure that medical supplies, emergency transportation, and a hospital are readily accessible. In addition to the usual cuts, scrapes, and crankiness that can pop up during any outing even with healthy children, the slightest fever, pain, or faintness in children whose immune systems are severely compromised requires immediate professional attention. A trip abroad increases the logistical complexity exponentially. And when you throw into the mix the fact that one of the children is a Palestinian who first has to obtain permission from the PA to cross into Israel to go on the trip and then has to make it through the usual stringent security screening at the airport in Lod, the efforts these young women have made to include Farhan are pretty impressive and a strong indicator of their devotion to him. They, too, have been able to see beneath the surface of Farhan's disfigurement, have been moved by his radiance and humanity, and have responded with an outpouring of compassion.

Farhan, who seems blissfully unaware of the politics and bureaucracy surrounding his trip, is so excited just to be part of it that throughout the trip he constantly posts photos of himself and the volunteers, thrilled to be sharing his experiences with everyone in our department. I can only imagine what the Europeans make of him. If only they knew how much love, hope, and humanity it took on the part of so many people to get him there.

I HAVE RETURNED TO ISRAEL with a fresh perspective, more attuned to nuances. As a result of my experiences in palliative care and in integrating its principles into my oncology practice, I start to become more at ease with ambiguity. This is evident as I become more comfortable accompanying my patients into the gray areas of prognostic uncertainty. But it's also evident in my own life. Process theology, which somehow accepts a divine force that is all-powerful and good, yet also, paradoxically, limited, somehow jibes with my own experience. I still don't feel totally Israeli and no longer feel completely American, but this bothers me less. In keeping with the principles of palliative care, I'm learning to embrace uncertainty as simply a part of living. With my initial small victories, I start to see how this plan to develop pediatric palliative care at Hadassah, and through it to define my career and place here in Israel, just might work.

11

Passages

M Y FIRST EXPOSURE TO THE DEATH of a patient
came during my third year of medical school, in Israel. It
was my first clinical rotation, which happened to be in internal
medicine. Tagging along with my mentor, a senior physician to
whom I had been assigned, on his morning rounds, I entered
the room of an elderly woman who was critically ill with an
antibiotic-resistant bacteria in her urinary system. The infection had spread throughout her frail body and was now wreak-
ing havoc on most of her vital organs. Observing her for a few
moments as she lay there unconscious, he said, "She's almost at
the end."

I scrutinized the woman's face, her breathing, the digital
readouts of the instruments, trying to understand what signs he
was so brilliantly interpreting. To me it seemed like voodoo, as
though through some dark art he was able to peer into her very
soul.

Assuming that with nothing more to do here we would

move on, I began to back away toward the door. But he surprised me by pulling a chair up to the bedside, sitting down, and taking one of the woman's limp hands in his own. I realize now that in addition to providing her with the comfort of a human touch, he was also probably assessing her pulse, feeling her skin growing cooler, judging the blood flow to her extremities. But at the time I saw it simply as a kind human gesture, all the more startling because, though so simple, it struck me as a profound part of what it means to be a healer. Even though I was only a medical student, I was already so lost in my books, so focused on physiology and on memorizing for tests, that I had forgotten for a moment what I was really training for.

"She has no family here," he said. "Never forget, if you accompany your patients only until the battle is lost and they are dying, if you abandon them at that point and leave them alone, you have done only part of your job, and not done it well. Your job is to accompany your patients until they are either better or safely on the other side."

What he was saying sounded vaguely familiar, but from a very different context. I was reminded of the funeral of my first grandparent to die, my maternal grandfather, when I was fifteen years old. At the graveside, after the few people in attendance had each thrown the traditional shovelful of earth into the open grave and I had moved off to the side, my father called me back.

"Take this," he said, keeping one shovel for himself and holding the other out for me. "We have to keep going until the grave is fully covered."

"Why?" I asked. "I already put some dirt in." I was still in the process of absorbing the loss of my grandfather and was in no hurry to participate in something so morbid.

"There's no one else here who can do it," he said. "The greatest thing you can do for him now as a grandson is to help me see to it that he is fully buried by us, his own family, and not just left for strangers to fill in the grave with a tractor."

It was incredibly difficult for me but I did it, of course, down to the last shovelful. And the experience stayed with me.

In the hospital room with my mentor and the dying woman, I sat down in a chair on the opposite side of the bed, not yet brave enough to hold her other hand but trying to take it all in. Except for the sounds of the three of us breathing, the room was still. As the minutes passed, the woman's breathing became slower, wetter, more ragged. And then, suddenly, it just stopped. She was gone. I had witnessed my first death.

After he checked that there was no pulse and that she was indeed deceased, my mentor notified the nurse in charge and quickly signed the death certificate. Then we moved on to the next patient on our rounds.

In one respect, which I didn't fully appreciate at the time, this was amazing. My mentor had demonstrated an incredibly valuable and, I would come to realize, incredibly difficult skill: how to be present during a death. But at the same time, I would later come to understand that he also displayed a poor adaptive response commonly seen in clinicians. He signed the certificate and moved on. That was it. To be fair, I don't know what was going on in his head, if he was hurting inside and saving it up until after work, or if he was truly so jaded and busy that he was unaffected by the death of his patient. All I saw as a student was that the patient was dead and we were expected to move on, with no comment or reflection on what had just occurred.

My understanding then and throughout my training was that with the departure of the doctor after the death of a patient, the nursing staff takes over. They would provide support to the patient's family and prepare the body to be moved to the hospital morgue. But as a medical student and later as a resident, I had no idea what any of this entailed. It's not part of a doctor's training. During my pediatric oncology fellowship the workload was so great and patient deaths so frequent, there never seemed to be time for me to even think about what happens to the body.

And, in any case, I soon realized that expressing concerns about these sorts of things was neither encouraged nor supported; in fact, I worried it would be perceived as a show of weakness.

At Hadassah, as a senior physician, I finally have more of an opportunity to observe what happens after the death of a patient. Because, in accordance with their religious traditions, most Jews and Muslims want to bury their deceased before sunset on the day of death (and because both religious traditions specify the avoidance of autopsies at all costs), things tend to move pretty quickly. Family members are allowed as much time as they need in the room with the child, but in the meantime, we fill out and register a death certificate with the hospital clerks, a process that always seems fast and efficient. Israel's bureaucracy is legendary, and Hadassah is generally no exception, but somehow the issuing of the death certificate always moves along quickly. It's almost as if there is a recognition that something terribly sad has occurred, and that the usual bureaucratic shenanigans of daily life at Hadassah should be set aside to allow a bereaved family to proceed swiftly and peacefully to their loved one's funeral.

Once the family has had some time alone in the room, we suggest that they step out so that we can clean the body. This is different from the ritual washing that the body will undergo once it has been transported to the appropriate burial society. But our washing and cleaning does take on its own special aura of ritual, and it's almost as if families recognize that there is something sacred about this final act that we carry out for our patients. Even the Haredi families, usually so protective of their own and alert to issues of modesty, allow us this special role. Death can be messy, even when peaceful. It may involve bleeding or the loss of fluids from any number of tubes and openings. As we clean the body with sponges and soapy water, we wipe away stains and clean any lacerations. We remove tubes, IVs, catheters, and tape, and even occasionally sew up wounds left after the removal of tubes and instruments, so that there is no ongoing spillage as the body is moved and so that the signs of disease and treatment are minimized. I've always felt that this allows us to return some dignity to the patient, to erase some of the ravages of the dying process.

The first time a nurse asked me if I would help, I hesitated. My job is done, my patient has passed away, why would I want to take part in something so, well, unpleasant? It was only later that I realized the invitation was not an attempt at off-loading work onto me but, rather, a respectful invitation. An honor, even. Being allowed to help clean my patient's body after his death, after my own treatments had failed, was an opportunity for me to provide one last act of kindness toward him. The patient, Dov, was a young man who had died of a progressive bone tumor. In the course of his treatment, one leg had been amputated. Despite that, the tumor had returned, spreading through his body and leaving the stump of his leg a swollen, rotting mass. The nurse caring for him very compassionately asked his family to wait outside as I went back into the room with her. Knowing what cancer can do to a person, my heart raced as I braced myself for what his exposed body might look like; in his final days I hadn't examined him thoroughly, not wanting to disturb him unnecessarily when the end was so close. She peeled back the sheets and, indeed, the stump and most of his lower body were engulfed and warped by the tumor. In several places the tumor had caused swelling and had even erupted from his body in fungus-like masses. I breathed through my mouth, afraid to smell the rotting flesh, and I focused on the nurse. She didn't flinch once. I followed her lead as she deftly, even lovingly, removed the tubes and wires still stuck to Dov. She wiped the sweat and blood from his motionless body, rolling him from right to left and then back again, to make sure nothing was missed. Together we lifted him onto a clean sheet, slipping the soiled ones out from underneath, and wrapped him so that only his head and face showed. The whole process seemed to transform him in just a few minutes from a victim of disease and its treatments to the picture of a young man finally at rest.

What surprised me most was that the process was also transformative for me. I felt a sense of fulfillment of my responsibility to this person who had been entrusted into my care. I was not in any way more reconciled with or any less sad about the death of my patient. But I had long sensed that just walking away from my patient once he had been declared dead left some part of the work unfinished. In this preparation of Dov's body, our staff carried out our final responsibilities to him, helping him complete his journey with dignity.

IN PEDIATRIC ONCOLOGY MOST PATIENT DEATHS do not come as a complete surprise. Usually we know when the odds are worsening and our patient is heading down a path with only one realistic ending. But actually predicting how much time remains for a patient is notoriously difficult, in contrast to what you might think based on the movies when the doctor so confidently and grimly predicts, "You've got six months to live." How long a terminally ill patient has left to live may depend on a number of factors, many of which are not under our control. This makes the timing of critical discussions about decision making and interventions incredibly important. At Hadassah, the point at which we see a child's disease progressing despite therapy is when we typically begin discussions with the parents about what to do should something happen suddenly. We need to know what sort of resuscitation efforts should be made if a patient stops breathing (in which case the team might consider intubation and mechanical ventilation) or if her heart stops beating (in which case the team might attempt cardiopulmonary resuscitation, or CPR). We refer to these sorts of discussions, the exploration of what the end might look like and what interventions make the most sense to a family, as advance care planning.

One issue that gets in the way of preparing for these possibilities is our Western culture's near-obsessive insistence on defining death as a discrete, identifiable moment. This may be a convenient way of viewing death for a number of reasons—for legal and administrative purposes, such as registering time of death and tracking data, or psychologically, as a way of quantifying death as a thing that we can then plan to stave off and "defeat." But death is not always so simple, so quantifiable. I now suspect that the first death I had witnessed in medical school, which I experienced as "here one minute, gone the next," was far more complex than I was able to appreciate at the time. The reason my mentor had us stay with his dying patient that day was probably that he saw that the dying process had already begun. All of my clinical experience since those early days as a student has only strengthened my understanding that death is a process and not just a moment in time.

Most religious and spiritual traditions seem to recognize this as well, and often do a better job of accommodating this reality than our own medical system does. Within the Jewish tradition, for example, there is a specific term, *goseis,* used to indicate a person who is what the medical profession calls "actively dying," who doctors believe has no more than hours or days left to live. According to kabbalistic traditions, the soul of the departed person remains present in the home during the week that the family sits shivah (which is one of the reasons the mirrors in the home are traditionally covered, so that the soul won't experience painful reminders that it no longer has a corporeal presence). There are non-Western traditions that incorporate this concept even more overtly into their beliefs surrounding death and dying. In the Tibetan Buddhist tradition, for example, when death appears to be approaching, holy men are brought to the bedside to chant prayers. Once the point is reached that we in the West would call "time of death," the holy men continue praying for three more days, which is considered to be a time of active transition for the spirit from one state to the next.

The inability, or unwillingness, to recognize death as a process inevitably leads to problems with having advance care planning discussions. Advance care planning doesn't mean "giving up" on a patient and stopping all forms of treatment. It simply means talking through with the patient and family members the what-ifs before a crisis ensues, and discussing in a relatively calm setting what procedures are most in line with the family's goals and religious or philosophical values. It doesn't mean that a patient has to stop hoping for a remission or even for a cure, or stop pursuing active treatments. It just means preparing for other, more likely possibilities. But however logical and reasonable this may seem in the abstract, pursuing this type of conversation is for many reasons often difficult for everyone—clinicians, patients, and families alike.

Clinicians are human beings, too, and they can sometimes engage in their own form of denial regarding signs of progressive disease or impending death in their patients. Or they may feel that this type of conversation is an acknowledgment of their own failure. They may worry that an unintended outcome of the conversation will be the loss of hope on the part of the patient and family. Whatever the reason, this is a difficult conversation for clinicians to initiate. They often avoid it by saying that the family "isn't there yet"; in other words, that the family isn't ready to face the possibility that their child will not be cured of her disease. But not having these conversations early enough may lead to unnecessary suffering by both the patient and her family, with death occurring amid a panicked, hurried mess of regrets over things left unsaid and comfort-oriented options not pursued. And all too often the family is, indeed, "there"; they're just waiting for the clinical team to open the discussion. The timing of advance care planning discussions can be tricky and, much like identifying a time of death, it can be difficult to identify a moment or trigger for starting the discussion.

There are better and worse ways to navigate these discussions. The clunkiest and possibly worst consists of a clinician laying out to parents the options of "doing everything" versus "just making the child comfortable." Unfortunately, this is sometimes how things are presented. It suggests, erroneously, that parents are faced with an either/or proposition: we will make your child feel comfortable, or we will use extraordinary measures to try to keep her alive. Worse yet, we place this unnecessary decision squarely on the ill-prepared shoulders of bewildered, grief-stricken parents. Alternatively, these conversations could happen in the context of a long-term relationship that has been established between the clinician and the family, during which a family's goals, values, and expectations have been thought through. In these instances, clinicians are able to provide guidance to parents on decision making and to suggest that, based on a family's beliefs or goals, there might be certain procedures or interventions that should or should not be done. This is often where a palliative care team can be helpful, especially if they have been introduced early enough and have developed a relationship with the child and her family. Our role is not to convince a family not to pursue interventions. It's simply to establish in advance, together with the family, what interventions are consistent with their goals and which are not. Sometimes this means not attempting resuscitation, and sometimes it means making that attempt, regardless of the clinicians' feeling that this would be futile.

Advance care planning is another realm where the rabbinic authorities in Israel play a major role, especially when it comes to the Haredi population. In an ideal world, communication between a patient's rabbi and the medical team would be seamless, everyone working together to explore goals, hopes, and fears in order to come up with a plan that is both medically and religiously or culturally appropriate for a given family. But in reality that sort of relationship rarely materializes. Our medical determinations and suggestions are more often sketchily conveyed by heartbroken parents to rabbis who can therefore have at best only a limited understanding of the patient's medical situation and prognosis. And so when we have advance care conversations with these families, what we most often hear is "The rabbi says that as long as there is life, we must do everything possible." Though it sounds definitive, there is an ambiguity in this response. Some clinicians will take this statement at face value and interpret it to mean that every attempt at resuscitation should be made no matter what. This will sometimes result in clinicians performing painful and pointless procedures on a dying child as weeping parents stand by, watching their child's final moments in horror, having not understood what they were signing on for. But sometimes clinicians will dig deeper, sensing that there are unresolved issues inherent in the statement. What is "everything"? they may ask. And when does "life" actually end? When is an action considered a reasonable intervention and when is it considered excessive and futile? When might an intervention actually fall into a category that is beyond "everything"? Often in my experience at Hadassah, when parents witness their child dying, when they see that the final moments are truly at hand, if we have developed a trusting relationship with them and have been engaging in these discussions over time, they tell us that attempting resuscitative efforts that are likely to be futile is not consistent with their values. In these situations, rather than asking for intubation and chest compressions, parents just want to hold their child and find meaning in those final moments of contact.

THERE IS, OF COURSE, another—and fortunately more common—end to some of our patients' stories: the successful completion of all planned therapy and, we hope, a long-term cure. But the reality is that no matter how well the therapy has worked, how successful the outcome, how optimistic the prognosis, this child's life and the lives of everyone in her immediate family have been changed forever. Uncertainty is not the exclusive province of those who are dying of cancer. Surviving cancer is physically, emotionally, and spiritually transformative in ways that can be positive or harmful, and sometimes even both. Clinicians often behave as though arriving at the last dose of planned chemotherapy is like crossing a finish line. We've won, you're cured, now go schedule your follow-up appointments in the outpatient clinic and come back sometime for a visit. It's perhaps not usually conveyed as curtly as that, but that's generally the gist of the conversation. This is certainly an important milestone, but it is by no means the end of the child's life as a patient. Follow-up appointments start out monthly, are later reduced to three or four times a year, and eventually become annual visits. They continue for years, because the odds of a recurrence of the disease are never zero and some of the long-term complications of chemotherapy can emerge at any time. But this is something that clinicians tend not to focus on in our final appointment with a patient and his family. Nor do we linger on the lasting psychological changes that the disease has made in all of their lives. We talk about how it takes time for kids to get back to their full energy level but that they'll get there. We remind them that their primary care doctor is now once again the child's regular pediatrician. But we have just spent months or years emphasizing how critical it is for them to bring their child in to us immediately, for even the slightest issue. They have meticulously followed lists of which foods are and are not okay, which medications must be taken in specific ways and at specific times. And now we send them off as though they can simply flip a switch and revert to their old lives. I've heard many families say that the two hardest days in their child's oncologic care were the day when they were first informed of their child's diagnosis, when their world was forever changed, and the day of discharge, when they had to leave the security of our clinic, with its treatment plans and charts, for the uncertainty of life "after" cancer. With the first sore throat or

runny nose after therapy has ended, parents often hurry back
to our clinic with their child, despite our reassurances that they
would be better served by their general pediatrician, because
the fear persists that every sore throat, every cough, every sore
muscle might herald the return of the disease. Even when children who are years off therapy, cured by every measure, come
back to visit us, somewhere in the small talk and the catching
up, between the embracing and the tears, there always seems to
be that desperate look in a parent's eyes that asks if everything
is really okay, if the child's cancer is really gone for good. I wonder if they see the same uncertainty reflected back in my own
face, because the truth is I don't know. No clinician does. I wish
I could help my patients and their families find meaning in the
emotional, spiritual, and physical trauma that they endured. But
I can't. I can only give them a hug, a pat on the back, or a few
carefully phrased encouraging words, and hope that this small
effort to be supportive helps them as they settle into lives that
have been irrevocably changed by what they have experienced.
There is now a field of medicine that specializes in long-term
follow-up of cancer survivors. They keep in touch with these
patients through the years, monitoring them for any medical
issues or other signs of trouble. I'm not myself an expert in this
field, but my experience in palliative care has made me more
sensitive to the necessity of this; it has certainly changed the
tenor of the discussions I now have with my patients and their
families as they return to life after cancer.

EXAMPLES OF THE TRANSFORMATIVE NATURE of near-
death experiences abound in the Bible, the Talmud, and the
Midrash (and can be found in the literature of other religious traditions as well). Because these texts are part of their national narrative, Israelis are better than most other Jews at using ancient
stories to make contemporary points. For example, even secular

Israelis are aware of the irony inherent in my given name. The biblical Elisha was a prophet, a disciple of the prophet Elijah. Elisha was also a wonder-worker—most famously when he brought back to life a boy who had died. As recounted in 2 Kings, Elisha utters a brief prayer and breathes into the boy's mouth, in one of the earliest recorded descriptions of medical resuscitation. My patients' families often jokingly ask me how my parents knew that I, too, would be a healer of children.

Many other biblical figures survive near-death experiences and are permanently transformed by them—Abraham, Ishmael, Isaac, Joseph, Jeremiah, Jonah, and Daniel, to name just a few. Their stories, though thousands of years old, still resonate for me in the lives of people here today, when the periodic outbreaks of violence result not only in death but also in frequent near-death experiences that carry their own special form of trauma. But what can Israelis and Palestinians do with their trauma? Just become more vengeful? More full of hate? Will they ever find a way to transform their anger into something that makes room for healing and that allows them to think about what life might look like here after all this fighting is done?

IT'S BEEN FOUR MONTHS since I've returned to Hadassah, and I've succeeded in getting donors to commit a significant amount of money for the development of a pediatric palliative care service here. At the same time, however, the rumblings about Hadassah's financial instability are becoming harder to ignore. In hindsight, I realize that a few of the people I had met with in the United States for advice had tried politely to warn me about the impending crisis, but either their warnings were too subtle or I was just so focused on my goal that I didn't want to hear them.

Encouraged by the commitment of funds, I push ahead and put together a more detailed document that lays out how the funds should be allocated, hoping that over the coming weeks I can start recruiting a team. But just when I've scheduled a meeting with Hadassah's director of operations, word begins to spread of an impending employees' strike, primarily over aggressive salary cuts that have just been announced. And it's not just cost-saving measures that are being discussed. The hospital is locked in negotiations with the government over ways to reduce a multimillion-dollar budget deficit that is actually calling Hadassah's very survival into question. The strike starts with the office workers and support staff but it quickly spreads, with the backing of the unions, to the nurses and the physicians. The salary cuts have an immediate impact on everyone. On top of that, there is a sense that the negotiations between Hadassah and the government, which have been dragging on for months, are going nowhere. No one expects the strike to last more than a few days, and the hope is that just a brief strike will provide the shock that the powers that be need to get moving toward a solution. But as the strike enters its second week, things begin grinding to a near-total halt. Two weeks may not sound like much time, but for a bustling hospital that normally works twenty-four hours a day to care for nearly a million patients a year, two weeks takes a huge toll on both the staff and the community. The emergency room and delivery rooms remain up and running, but every other department starts to look utterly abandoned. Even in the middle of the day the gleaming new lobby feels dead and empty, echoing with the footsteps of the few staff members still coming in. Operating rooms function only on an emergency basis, and each case has to be vetted by a union committee before the staff is permitted to prepare for a procedure. Among the cases that have to be vetted are children from our department who have been scheduled for surgery.

"Why is this an emergency?" the committee asks when I petition for a young man to have a tumor removed from his face. "Will he die if the tumor isn't removed this week?"

How to answer that? The tumor isn't growing so quickly that its immediate removal could be considered a matter of life and death, but at the same time who really knows what could happen down the road? The patient has been getting weeks of chemotherapy, and based on his protocol he is now due for surgery. His parents know this. He knows this. How can I tell them that he has to spend more time with this ever-present threat in his body while Hadassah and the government argue over shekels? And if the tumor returns at some future date, how would we ever know whether one or two cancer cells had spread while his surgery was delayed, leading to the disease's recurrence? We're not alone in this. Every clinician in the hospital is faced with the same dilemma. How do we simultaneously support the strike and our patients?

Each day turns into a struggle to make sure we're providing the best care possible for our patients. Some families move their medical care elsewhere. There are rumors that the emergency rooms in other local hospitals are becoming overwhelmed as people intentionally avoid Hadassah. We continue to receive new patients in pediatric oncology, but even here we feel the effects of the strike. Under Mickey's leadership we try to create a safe bubble for our patients and their families, and we make an effort not to speak about the strike where they might overhear us. But there is no way to completely ignore what is going on. Due to the skeleton staffing in radiology and other diagnostic labs, we have to send some of our patients to other institutions for scans and ask them to bring the results back to us on discs. These are difficult conversations to have. Parents flat-out ask me if they should just transfer their child's care to another hospital, if the level of care here is being affected by the strike. I reassure them that we are still delivering the same quality of care as we always have been and then I hand them a referral for an MRI at another hospital, aware of the absurd contradiction between my words and my actions. I don't think we are necessarily endangering our patients, but I worry that this won't be true if the strike goes on for much longer.

On top of our anxieties about patient care is the stress of managing our personal finances during the crisis. Email announcements about the strike and the hospital's finances arrive almost daily. One day it's that there is no pay at all, one day it's that pay is reduced, one day it's that pay will be withheld but will be repaid at some future point (a future that nobody seems certain even exists). Compared to some of my colleagues, I am lucky. I have some savings, and I have a family that I know I can fall back on if I run out of money. Others are in much more dire financial circumstances. I listen, horrified, to colleagues talking about cutting back on essentials as they try to figure out how they are going to put food on the table for their kids, how they are going to pay for medicine. It's almost impossible for me to believe that the jewel in Israel's healthcare system has arrived at this point.

After two weeks, the strike ends and negotiations among the hospital, the government, the unions, and the Hadassah Women's Zionist Organization of America begin to move forward. But the air of crisis continues and the financial issues don't seem to improve. Funds remain frozen. Money from grants and donations, including mine, can be used only with permission from the top administrators. Rumors begin to circulate that those funds have, in fact, been used, or have been reallocated, or, most ominously, have been "lost." When I try to find out where the donations I had brought in have gone, I can't get a straight answer. Half the people I ask tell me the funds are still in the United States and haven't yet been transferred over from the Hadassah Women's Zionist Organization; the other half insist that they are safely in the hospital's coffers. Either way, the bottom line is that they are now officially out of my hands. And because I have no formal, binding agreement with the hospital administration regarding the allocation of the money I had brought in, I have lost all control over it.

I'm not even sure where to direct my anger. In trying to figure out how the hospital has gotten into this mess, fingers point
in every direction. Some blame poor investment choices, some
point to mismanagement on the part of the government, others
to mismanagement on the part of the hospital. My sense is that
it was probably a combination of all these factors.

I sit through more than a few meetings with Hadassah's physicians and administrators, during which the depth of the crisis
we are in is made terrifyingly clear. There will be layoffs, salary
reductions, reallocations of resources. The Israeli government
might assist in bailing us out, the Hadassah Women's Zionist
Organization of America will help as much as they can (as victims of Bernard Madoff, they have their own financial problems),
and, hopefully Hadassah will be restored to fiscal stability. If that
fails, there are rumors of a buyout, that the hospital could be
taken over by one of the other HMOs. As I listen to all this, I
know, even without being told, that my dream of a pediatric palliative care program here is just about dead. And, even worse, I'm
left wondering how secure my job and my future as an attending
physician in the Pediatric Hematology-Oncology Department
really is.

12

Abandonment

THE NEWS SPREADS SLOWLY. At first there are just rumors and gossip, a whiff of tension in the air, and then the official reports on the news programs confirm what by now everyone already knows. I'm at home in Jerusalem on a warm June evening in 2014, about four months after Hadassah's financial crisis went public. News alerts begin to pop up on my phone about large numbers of soldiers and police gathering in a field outside an Arab village near Hebron, in the West Bank. There is little doubt about what that means. Three Jewish teenagers had been kidnapped three weeks earlier while hitchhiking near a West Bank settlement. The only question now is whether the soldiers are gathering to launch a rescue mission or to retrieve the boys' dead bodies. Reports quickly confirm the latter and, even more heartbreaking, that the boys had most likely been killed very shortly after they were abducted by Palestinians with ties to Hamas.

A palpable tension had descended upon Jerusalem when the

boys first went missing, a combination of anger and fear that
began to seep into everyday life in the city and into our department as well. After months of trying to shelter our patients from
the financial chaos at Hadassah, the added burden of coping
with one more crisis is becoming too much for us to handle. If
the bubble in which we all try to live and work does not exactly
burst, it does, unmistakably, start to deflate. The veneer of calm
and safety begins to wear off.

Although the strike is over, the financial problems at Hadassah persist. Support staff and clinicians continue to leave, some
voluntarily and some not. Many more clinicians grumble threats
about leaving; the ones who actually quit are unwilling to risk
their careers or their families' well-being on what increasingly
feels like a sinking ship. I try to cling to a naive hope that the
funds I had brought in will insulate me from the crisis and allow
me to develop my palliative care program regardless of any aus-
terity cuts the hospital has to make. But, at the same time, I am
talking to other hospitals in Israel about my project, recognizing
that at least for now the likelihood of my making progress at
Hadassah is increasingly close to zero. In many respects I have
taken an approach to my own life that I learned through my
work in palliative care: hope for the best, but prepare for the
worst, all the while somehow muddling through the grayness of
uncertainty. If I leave Hadassah, my preference would be to find
a job at another Israeli hospital, especially because my entire
family is now here. But as I explore options with other medical
centers, I can't escape the feeling that they are more interested
in my American donors than in my project.

"Would your existing donors be willing to redirect their
funds to another hospital?" one administrator asks slyly.

Another tells me after a series of exploratory meetings, "First,
you tell us if you're coming, then we can talk about the details
of the position. I don't want to go through the whole process
of thinking about how to structure a job that you might not

accept." For me, that's a nonstarter; I'm done with securing my future with handshakes and vague promises.

And so I also begin to look at positions that might be available in the United States. This is, to some extent, influenced by the fact that I've met a woman who has changed how I think about my identity and my future. Sasha is a bit of a global citizen. She grew up in both the United States and Europe, and none of her passports seem to quite match her accent. Though I meet her in Israel, she's wide open to journeying wherever life may take her. Whereas I had always placed such an emphasis on location, pinning my identity and ideology to geography, Sasha seems to derive strength from her willingness to move and to change. I'm beginning to see that geography might not be the most important determinant of who we are. Sasha has shown me that there can be beauty in uncertainty, that sometimes (as I should have recognized through my work experience) uncertainty can also mean opportunity. Though we both prefer to remain in Israel, I am now thinking about a future with a wife and children, and I feel that I must explore options that include leaving Israel for a more secure job in the States.

THREE DAYS AFTER THE MURDERED BOYS have been buried, Israel is rocked by another event unimaginable in its horror. A teenage Palestinian boy is kidnapped from a street in East Jerusalem, beaten, and burned to death by three Israeli Jews. The murder is widely condemned throughout Israel—the families of the three murdered Israeli teens publicly express their condolences to the family of the murdered Palestinian boy, and several government officials visit the mourning family—but the tension in Jerusalem escalates beyond anything I'd ever seen there. Gangs of right-wing Jewish thugs begin roaming the streets at night, harassing and beating any Arabs unfortunate enough to cross their path. They also take to intimidating left-wing demonstrators trying to advocate for calm. I am appalled by what is happening, and I retreat further into work. My life exists within two bubbles: evenings at home with Sasha, since we now rarely venture out after dark, and days in the Pediatric Hematology-Oncology Department, where, perpetually focused on the dramas unfolding in the lives of our patients, we try to ignore what is happening outside.

The fact that it is Ramadan adds another layer of complexity and sadness to a rapidly deteriorating situation. I can see that my Muslim colleagues at Hadassah are quieter than usual, more withdrawn. Observant Muslims who work during Ramadan always appear more tired as the day wears on and the fast takes its toll, especially toward the end of the month. For their sake we try to schedule meetings in the morning hours, when they may still feel energized by the predawn *suhur* meal. But this year the fatigue seems to be more pronounced, as everyone's energies are additionally sapped by the ongoing tensions. Every night angry people take to the streets: Jewish right-wingers looking for trouble, Muslim youths throwing stones, and observers of Ramadan who just want to get some fresh air after their evening banquet. It's a mix that seems primed for an explosion.

I had become accustomed to jogging in the early morning, before sunrise. I would run along the old Ottoman-era train tracks in the southwestern part of the city, which had recently been converted to a promenade and bike path. My favorite section, not far from where I live, is where the tracks follow a path between the West Jerusalem neighborhood of Katamon and the East Jerusalem Arab neighborhood of Beit Safafa, where Fatma lives.

But with the recent tensions I grow increasingly uncomfortable on my jogs. Beit Safafa seems more alive than usual in the early morning hours, as people wake for the predawn meal. I feel guilty for thinking this way, but with all of the violence going on I worry about what might happen if I am caught alone mid-run by a group of young men from the village looking to vent their anger. Beit Safafa, which I have visited many times, now feels alien and threatening. I ask Fatma if I need to worry about this, and after thinking about it for a moment she makes a face I understand to mean that it's not worth looking for trouble. I consider jogging after work, while it's still light out.

And then, as if things couldn't get any worse, rockets start coming down on us from Gaza. At first it's just an increase in the usual short-range fire—mortars and small rockets that for the most part strike areas in Israel that are close to the border with Gaza. The uptick is noticeable enough to make people in places like Jerusalem and Tel Aviv pay attention but limited enough in range so that we can pretend to be unaffected. Then the longer-range rockets start—the ones aimed at areas farther up Israel's coast and into southern Israel. Israel's Iron Dome defense system destroys most of the rockets before they can land, and with each thwarted attack that has traveled deeper inside Israel than the preceding one, there is a sense that this has got to be the farthest they will dare go. We soon realize how wrong we are.

The first air-raid siren to go off in Jerusalem comes one evening when I am home alone, curled up with a book on my couch. For a moment I think it must be some weird ambulance siren, but then I realize what's going on. With no steel-and-concrete-reinforced "safe room" in my apartment, I quickly take shelter in the bathroom, which is the room closest to the center of the building and the place I figure is least likely to take a direct hit from a rocket. I crouch down (as though crouching would make any difference if a rocket actually did land on my apartment), listening to the wailing siren, not sure what to expect. It's a strange feeling to know that a couple of minutes ago someone about sixty miles away fired a rocket that is now in flight on a trajectory controlled only by the laws of physics and possibly headed for my apartment building. I hear the unmistakable *boom* of a warhead exploding in the distance and take a deep breath.

I emerge shaken but relieved from my completely inadequate hiding place.

As I pull out of the Hadassah parking lot the next afternoon, another siren goes off. I keep driving for a full minute, not wanting to seem like a coward and not sure what the etiquette is for responding to an air-raid siren while in a moving vehicle. Then I realize that all the other cars on the road have pulled over to the side and their occupants have left their cars to take cover. I pull over, too, and join some people in a shallow drainage ditch that, again, affords little realistic protection. I can hear what sounds like a jet engine, and in the cloudless sky above the hospital I see what looks like a small plane flying up from the south and passing over the hospital. As it flies over our heads I wonder if it's a military plane, and I hope the pilot realizes that there's a rocket coming in. He seems to be flying pretty low, and all I can think is how horrible it would be if he took a direct hit. From over the hill behind us, two small streaks of fire arc toward the plane, and just when they seem to be about to strike it they explode, one after the other. There is a stronger, thundering explosion, as what I thought was a plane but is actually the incoming rocket blows up, having been intercepted by those two Iron Dome missiles. People climb out of their hiding places, smiling and pointing skyward. Someone applauds. I couldn't even if I wanted to; my hands are shaking. It's one thing to see this sort of thing when you're in the army, even on reserve duty, when you're part of a fighting force that has plans in place for when things like this happen. It's another thing altogether to confront an incoming rocket when you're alone in your car driving home after a long day of work.

I resume my drive home, stopping first at the supermarket, where people are shopping as though nothing has happened. That's the way it is here. Though there was just a rocket attack a few miles away and there could be another one at any moment, for now the task at hand is to go about our lives, pick up the kids, and buy the groceries for dinner.

Then the real war starts.

As we watch the ramp-up of Hamas rocket fire and Israeli air strikes, reports emerge that troops are being mobilized in the south. We all try to convince ourselves that neither side really wants this to happen, that there must be back-channel negotiations going on to find a way out without anyone losing face. Rumors spread that reservists are being called up. I get a call from the army canceling the training exercises that had been planned for my unit this month. Nothing to worry about, the coordinating officer says, it would just be hard to do drills with the troop buildup in the south going on. But stay available, she throws in casually at the end of our conversation, we'll call when we need you.

Both of the pediatric oncology fellows in our department get calls the next day to report to their reserve units, and we scramble to reorganize our schedules to make up for their absence. I feel a twinge of fear and, surprisingly, a pang of jealousy. My reserve unit operates in the same area as theirs. Does that mean I, too, will get called up? Will I actually see open combat? The fellows appear calm as they tidy up before leaving, but you can see the concern; we are all fully aware of the fact that some people who go off to war don't come home.

DROR IS A FOURTEEN-YEAR-OLD PATIENT in our department who is in his final days, if not hours, of dying from a progressive sarcoma. As always, it's difficult to predict exactly when it will happen. His brother, who is serving with one of the units that is now encircling Gaza, has been released for a few hours to come here to say goodbye. Dror's parents remain planted at his bedside, afraid to step away for even a moment, but Dror's brother pulls Mickey and me out into the hallway. With tears in his eyes, he tells us in a low voice that his unit has just received the order to prepare to enter Gaza. His friends are now pulling their gear together for an invasion set to begin that very night. What should he do? he asks us. Stay here at his dying brother's bedside and abandon his comrades? Or return to his unit and abandon his dying brother? I have no idea how to answer. Part of me is still taken aback by the fact that he has just divulged to us a serious military secret, and that if it turns out to be true, Israel will be well into a ground invasion by the morning. Mickey's own son has been sent to the border with his reserve unit, and I can't figure out how he appears so calm and able to focus on work. Say your goodbyes to Dror, Mickey says, and go back to your unit. Your brother is going to die whether you are here or not. But if you don't go back to your unit and someone there gets hurt or killed, you'll never forgive yourself. Dror's brother nods and goes back into the room. I just stand there. This is not something they teach you in medical school or something you are likely to encounter during a fellowship in New York or Boston.

When I leave work later that day, Dror's brother and two of his friends happen to get into the elevator with me. As we exit to the parking lot, the sun already starting to sink behind the hills, I take his hand and tell him to be careful. He nods and gives me a wry smile. I'm still trying to wrap my head around the fact that in a few hours he and thousands of other soldiers will be at the front in a full-scale ground war.

As it turns out, the incursion into Gaza doesn't happen that night. I cling to the hope that it's a sign that both sides are busy negotiating their way out of this. But then one night just a few days later, it is suddenly under way. A barrage of rockets launched by Hamas at Tel Aviv—where I happen to be having dinner with my parents and Sasha—is the first indication that something is happening, but we are soon watching on television footage of drifting illumination flares over Gaza, a sure sign that our infantry are on their way in. The ground war—this one called Operation Protective Edge—has begun.

It's hard for me to understand how our department is still managing to function. As we continue to care for our patients, we are also dealing with the day-to-day effects of Hadassah's financial crisis, the violence in the streets of Jerusalem, and, now, an all-out war.

"Where do we move the kids in the event of an air-raid siren?" I ask, half-joking, since I know there's really nowhere to go. There is a small "reinforced room" near our offices that's designed to function as a bomb shelter, but it's been converted to a storage room for patient charts. It's so loaded with file cabinets and shelves full of folders that we've often joked that if we ever have to take shelter there, at least we'll have something to read. But now, with rockets flying over Jerusalem, it isn't such a joke. We have children here who are so sick, so frail, so dependent on machines, that even moving them around in their beds for a quick daily wash can be risky. Bringing them down to Radiology for a scan or to the operating room might require several people, moving slowly and carefully so as not to pull out any tubes or disconnect any equipment. So how are we supposed to move two dozen sick kids to safety in a matter of minutes?

If there's a siren, Mickey explains, any child who can get out of bed on his own or be easily carried by a family member should be moved into the hallway, which at least is away from the windows. The children with more complicated needs who would not be able to make it into the hallway should be taken into their bathroom if at all possible, where there are also no windows. But we all know that in the event of an air raid, there is no way we will be able to get every child to a safer place. And, anyway, if a rocket hits one of the rooms, how much of a difference will it really make to be a few feet away, in the bathroom or the hallway? For the most part, we just have to hope and pray that nothing actually hits us.

WHILE ALL OF THIS IS GOING ON, I receive a job offer from a hospital in New York. It's as though I'm being tested. The job description is essentially everything that I had hoped to do at Hadassah: setting up and running a pediatric palliative care service at a well-known and highly respected teaching hospital. In contrast to Hadassah, they are offering me job security, a dedicated staff, and funding. The only problem, of course, is that it's not in Israel, which was such an important part of my dream. This wasn't supposed to be just about establishing a pediatric palliative care service; it was about doing it *here*. And having been back and forth one time too many over the past few years, I'm not all that thrilled about pulling up stakes and relocating yet again.

I'm really not sure what to do and so, looking for advice, I share my news with some colleagues at Hadassah. One says that it sounds like a great offer but that if he were in my shoes there is no way he would go. Israel is home, he says, going for my weak spot, and the noblest type of service is to stay here and help our own people. Others disagree, saying that if they had received an offer like mine they would take it, and that I should worry about my own career and well-being first.

As I'm debating what to do, I receive a notice from the Health Ministry in response to my recent application for a certificate recognizing my advanced palliative care training. There are no fellowships in Israel specific to pediatric palliative care. Given my training and work experience in Boston, at this moment in time I am literally the most highly trained pediatric palliative care clinician in the entire country. And yet, in a reply that reminds me of what I had to go through to get my medical license when I first arrived here, they tell me that they don't feel that my training and work experience in the United States are sufficient and that they'd like me to reapply in the future with "further documentation." Where in the world I'm supposed to get further training or documentation isn't at all clear. If I didn't know better, I'd say someone at the Ministry of Health is doing this on purpose.

One of the top administrators at Hadassah asks to meet with me, knowing that I am considering returning to the United

States. He wants to see if he can convince me to stay on. Increasingly cynical about the inner workings of Hadassah, I can't help but think that they are more worried about losing the donor money that I've brought in than about losing me. He admits that the institution cannot give me any guarantees about the palliative care program, or even about access to the funds that I've raised. That pretty much decides it for me. When I tell him that I don't feel I can plan my future based on vague promises, he nods. Realizing that I mean to leave, he pauses and, in a complete shift of tone, says that truth be told, he would tell his own child to do the same thing.

I walk out of his office, my mind made up, but I'm surprised to find that I feel even worse than I felt going in. Why do I feel such guilt? Or is it just disappointment in the death of a dream? In pediatric oncology we often use the unfortunate term "abandonment" to refer to situations where parents of children undergoing treatment stop bringing their kids in for appointments. This is a particular challenge in developing countries, where the financial and social burdens placed on families with a sick child may simply be too much for them to bear. It's not that the parents don't love their child or don't care enough. It may just be that they have stopped believing in the possibility of a cure, and have started worrying more about the toll the treatment is taking on their child and on the rest of their family. Though we refer to it as "abandonment," it might be fairer to view it as parents making a difficult choice in an impossible situation. The palliative care clinician in me says that in these situations the challenge should be to improve the medical system, to understand the needs and concerns of the family, to work within the family's value system to provide better choices, and to improve infrastructure to make care more easily accessible for those who need it.

I mull this over as I wonder if I am abandoning my country. I find myself forced to choose between pursuing my dream in a place that seems consistently to foil my best intentions—a country that has sapped my finances and whose national policies seem to be increasingly set on a path contrary to everything I believe in—and building my career as a palliative care clinician in an environment that will be supportive, both financially and culturally, where I can develop my skills and secure my future but that doesn't feel like "home."

I know I should stop taking this so personally, that I should accept that the system and the country owe me nothing. But it's only human to feel that, having been prepared to give so much, I should receive some sort of affirmation of the value of what I have tried to accomplish over the past seven years. What I'm feeling is the pain of unrequited love. It's not that the system is against me, it's that the system simply doesn't care.

THE WAR RAGES ON, and I'm on call one Saturday, doing morning rounds. Ronit, a fourteen-year-old girl who has been under our care for years with a slowly progressing sarcoma, has been deteriorating over the past few weeks, and she now seems to be very close to the end. She is asleep most of the time. Her face is tinged a faint blue, her nose flaring and chest heaving, trying to pull in as much oxygen as possible past the advancing tumors in her lungs. I think of the Arab father and son with whom I had sat in this very room during the war between Israel and Gaza back in 2009. The memory brings a sad feeling of déjà vu but also a strange sense of security. Here in this room, with no sounds but Ronit's quiet, labored breathing, the oxygen whispering through the nasal prongs, the occasional beeping of pumps, there is a comforting familiarity. In my heart I have, of course, wished for a different outcome for Ronit, just as we hope for a different outcome for all of our patients who don't survive, but I know what is coming and I accept its inevitability. In this room I can try momentarily to forget everything going on outside and focus on just this space, this one life. Although I know I cannot cure Ronit, there is still so much I can do: relieve her symptoms, maintain a comfortable environment, oversee her and her parents' experience of what is happening. With all of the violence and insanity outside, with all of the uncertainty about what condition the hospital will find itself in when the financial dust settles and what condition Israel will find itself in when a cease-fire is finally declared, in this room, at least, is something that, if not totally comprehensible, is at least recognizable.

The nurse caring for Ronit is a young Israeli Arab woman. Maryam and I go into Ronit's room together after morning rounds to assess her breathing and comfort and to make a plan for the day, trying to anticipate any sudden emergencies that might arise. Ronit is lying in bed with her head propped up on a mound of pillows, her eyes closed. Her parents have taken advantage of the quiet to slip outside for a cigarette, so the two of us are alone at Ronit's bedside, watching as she takes one difficult breath after another.

Slowly, as though waking from a dream, Ronit opens her eyes and looks at us. After a few moments, she raises her thin arms out in front of her.

"You want help sitting up?" We are both guessing, because she is too weak to speak.

Ronit barely manages a nod. Maryam goes around to the opposite side of the bed and we each take one of her hands, placing our other hand under her for support. We gently lift her up while adjusting the head of the bed upward, until she is sitting up and appears comfortable. As we both start to step back, Ronit twists her hands and locks them onto our forearms.

"What?" We try to guess, using yes/no options so that she can just nod. "Higher? Lower? Another pillow?"

But she doesn't respond, doesn't even nod. She just grips our arms as she stares at us. Somehow this frail child manages slowly to pull us in so that we are eventually crouching by her side, holding her hands. We kneel like that in silence, for what feels like many minutes, the three of us forming a silent, frozen tableau.

We leave the room when Ronit's parents return, knowing that in her own way she has just told us goodbye. My rounds completed, I go home. There's no way to be sure how long this might go on, but Ronit appears to be comfortable and her parents are with her, so I leave the hospital with instructions to call me if anything changes. I know that I can return quickly if need be, but I also suspect that it is the last time I will see her alive. And, indeed, barely an hour later Ronit quietly passes away.

By the time I get the call and return to the hospital, the nurses are in the midst of washing Ronit's body. I slip into the room for a moment for one last silent farewell. Orderlies arrive to take her down to the morgue to await the arrival of the members of the burial society at end of the Sabbath, and her family goes home to begin preparations for the funeral and for shivah. Rather than head right home again I sit in the break room with Maryam. The intensity of that shared goodbye, combined with the war that is raging outside and the fact that it's a weekend, seem to grant us permission to say things that would not normally be said at work.

"Elisha," she says, "I don't know what I'm doing. This is crazy. Everything we're doing here, this whole situation doesn't make sense."

"I know," I say, not sure if she is referring to the fact that a child has just died, that the hospital is crumbling, or that the country is at war. "Everything feels surreal lately."

"No, you don't understand," she says angrily. "I'm here, caring for this dying Jewish girl, even washing her body after she dies. And meanwhile Israeli planes and soldiers are killing my friends and relatives not far from here. And who is caring for them?"

It takes a moment for me to register what she is talking about. What friends and relatives? I had always bought into the narrative that Israeli Arabs are a people separate and distinct from Palestinian Arabs. How foolish that seems when you take a moment to think about the fact that Israeli Arabs obviously have relatives and friends in the West Bank and Gaza. As I'm sitting here feeling conflicted about my own allegiances, wondering if I should stay at Hadassah, take that job in New York, or join the fighting in Gaza, this woman, grounded in the land in a way I never will be, struggles with her own conflicted identity. I came to Israel because I thought this was where my questions about identity would be resolved. But they've only become more complex during the time I've spent here. And the saddest thing is that the self-styled vigilantes who murder teenagers, the terrorists who fire rockets into population centers, the fundamentalists who illegally appropriate land—they are the ones who seem most certain of their identities, and they seem to be the ones driving the narrative.

But despite the sadness of this moment, sitting here with Maryam I catch a glimpse of the Israel I had hoped for and that I still hope for: an Israeli Muslim and an American-Israeli Jew, each in our differently accented Hebrew, bound together in caring for these children and in wishing things were different.

AS THE WAR ENTERS ITS THIRD WEEK, I find myself more and more conflicted. Yes, something has to be done about all those rockets Hamas has been raining down on us, but every day brings news reports of Gaza civilians, including children, being killed because of mistaken missile coordinates or because Hamas has set up rocket launchers a few feet away from their homes. While I'm roughhousing one day with my three-year-old niece, she thinks she's being funny when she attempts to escape my clutches by shouting, "Air raid! Everyone run quickly to the shelter!" I can't believe that this has become part of everyday conversation for a kid. She doesn't yet understand what these words mean, how afraid she really should be. Her six-year-old brother, a bit wiser, understands that the sirens and the boom of intercepted rockets means that "bad people" are trying to hurt him. "Are you going to go with the army to stop them?" he asks me solemnly, not fully understanding what he is saying, either. And a part of me aches to say yes, yes, I'm going, I'm a part of this, and we will fix it and everything will be all right.

WE ARE HAVING A STAFF MEETING in Mickey's office when the father of one of our patients, a ten-year-old boy from Gaza with a recurrent muscle tumor, calls the social worker's cellphone. Kareem can't breathe, he says. The army has been shelling the buildings on either side of their home, and he doesn't know what to do. He wants our help in getting his son back to Hadassah.

We debate among ourselves. It's possible that Kareem is having a panic attack from the fighting around him, but it's also possible that he's experiencing shortness of breath because of his advancing tumor. We advise Kareem's father to get him to the closest hospital in Gaza; it's too dangerous to try to get him out through the fighting, and if he really is experiencing the effects of his disease, once he's in a hospital we can appeal through the proper channels to have him transferred to Hadassah.

I look at Mickey. "How does God allow this to happen?" I ask, rhetorically. The others in the room look down, avoiding eye contact.

With a sad smile, the director rubs his face. "Dr. Waldman," he says slowly, "don't you realize by now that we're all on our own down here? That nobody up there is looking out for us?"

I don't answer.

Later that afternoon I hear on the news that the army has shelled the upper floors of a hospital in Gaza after being fired upon from that location. I wonder if that's where Kareem's father took him. I wonder if they are still alive.

As it turns out, Kareem remained at home, and a few days later, during a lull in the fighting, his ever-resourceful mother manages to bring him in from Gaza for a checkup. Aside from his visibly progressing tumor, he seems to be doing well and is at least comfortable. We take some blood tests and give his mother a new supply of his oral chemotherapy. While we are waiting for the test results, Kareem sits quietly off to one side in the waiting area. A group of soldiers have come to distribute candy to the kids as an act of community service, and I see one of them offer Kareem a packet of sweets. He takes it, nodding his thanks but barely looking up.

How odd it must be for him, being handed candy by a soldier from the same army that has just leveled his neighborhood, leaving hardly a building intact. Kareem's mother is standing in the hall near our offices, arguing with the head administrative assistant. She's gesturing furiously at pictures on her mobile phone that show the rubble where buildings had stood only a few days ago. The administrator is countering with video clips from foreign news services that show Hamas militants firing rockets from alongside civilian buildings. I'm pretty sure that neither woman will ever be able to convince the other to see it her way.

AS THE THIRD WEEK OF FIGHTING draws to a close, I go for a late afternoon jog along the train tracks. The sun is just beginning to set, and there are plenty of people about. I've been packing all day and getting ready for my return to New York, all while keeping close track of the news. I need to get out for a run, just to clear my head.

The setting sun bathes the valley in gold, and there is a strong scent of dry rosemary in the hot wind. I can almost forget everything that is going on around us, and for a moment it feels like the Jerusalem I remember from the summers I spent here as a kid.

At the point where the neighborhoods of Katamon and Beit

Safafa are closest, divided just by the old train tracks, the Hand in Hand organization runs a bilingual school where Arab and Jewish children from the Jerusalem area learn together. The building is located on the Katamon side of the tracks, to my right as I jog down the valley. As I approach the school I see a huge white banner made of bedsheets hanging from the side of the building that faces Beit Safafa. On it is written in black paint, in Hebrew and Arabic, WE REFUSE TO BE ENEMIES.

I stop running, overwhelmed by the power of this simple proclamation—the beauty, the majesty, even, of this handmade sign and the message it is sending across the valley. This evidence that there are still some sane people in the city gives me a small measure of comfort.

The next day I can barely wait to show Fatma a picture of the banner I had taken with my phone. I am excited to share with her this glimmer of hope.

Fatma looks at the picture and sighs. Yes, she says, that's the school my kids go to. An identical banner had been hung on the other side of the building as well, she tells me, on the side that faces Katamon. They had to take it down after a day because someone had spray painted DEATH TO ARABS across it.

I want to cry.

Mickey looks exhausted, as usual. He's been run down by months of trying to maintain the protective bubble around our department. But he appears to be less tense today than he has been lately. He tells us that he was up all night, having received a call from the army last evening telling him that his son was being taken from his unit to a hospital in southern Israel to be treated for dehydration. Mickey drove down to the hospital in the middle of the night to pick his son up and bring him home. He had been offered several days' leave at home to recuperate, but he refused, insisting on taking just a day to recover before returning to his unit.

"So," Mickey says, sighing, "we slept well last night, after getting our son home. And we will sleep well tonight, while he is home, and tomorrow is a new day."

"How can you be so calm?" Fatma asks.

"What other choice do we have but to hope?" he replies. "If we stop hoping we have nothing, and then all is lost."

Epilogue

I'M SURPRISED BY HOW REASSURINGLY FAMILIAR New York feels. Sasha and I have been here for two months, and I'm slowly settling into my new job at New York–Presbyterian Hospital but still aching over the move. I feel like I've just performed surgery on myself—sliced into my body, removed an organ, and am now waiting for the incision to heal. The air-raid sirens are gone, but they have been replaced by sirens from the fire station across the street from our apartment on Manhattan's Upper West Side. One of the trucks has a siren that sounds uncannily like the Israeli air-raid sirens, with that same low, slow windup, and we still jump reflexively when we hear it. But with each day that passes, thinking about Jerusalem hurts less and New York begins to seem more and more like home.

New York–Presbyterian serves a large population of Hasidic Jews, and it initially seems odd to me to encounter them in upper Manhattan. Back in Jerusalem I had been very aware of our differences and the gulf between us, but here I feel as though we

share a secret bond, and treating their kids brings back fond
memories, frustrations notwithstanding, of my Haredi patients
and their families at Hadassah. Shortly after I start my job I am
asked to do a palliative care consultation for a four-year-old
Hasidic girl in intensive care. In addition to her current bout of
influenza, Esther has a number of congenital anomalies related
to a poorly understood genetic disorder, and I've been asked to
explore and clarify goals of care with her family. The primary
care team reports that her parents have tentatively agreed to
meet with me.

That afternoon I go into Esther's room to meet with her
father, who is alone with her. A burly man in a long black coat
and fur hat, with a thick beard and *payos,* he looks just like the
Haredim in Jerusalem's Orthodox neighborhoods. I feel weirdly
transported back to Hadassah. Esther's father is standing between
the bed and the window, rocking rhythmically as he prays from a
book of Psalms. I introduce myself and explain that I'm the doctor who has been referred by Esther's primary care physician to
help them sort out some of the details of her care.

"Ve don't need you," he says in a thick Yiddish accent, barely
looking up from his book. "Ve're okay."

I adopt my warmest, most nonthreatening voice and offer
to come by and talk at any time, but he shoos me away. There's
nothing to be gained by pressing the issue, so I say goodbye with
a promise to stop by again just to see how things are going in
case he changes his mind.

I stop by Esther's room daily but never manage to catch
either parent there, only volunteers from their Hasidic community who take turns maintaining a constant vigil at her bedside.
Then, passing by one evening on my way out, I see her father,
his back to me, hunched over his book of Psalms as though he
hadn't moved since our last encounter. I pause and, sensing my
presence, he turns. He looks up at me for a split second, quickly
looks down at his book, and then just as quickly looks back up
and gestures gruffly with his hand.

"Come in," he mutters. I smile brightly, ready to launch my charm offensive, and step into the room.

Swaying from side to side as though lost in prayer, he keeps his head down, eyes locked on the book, furtively glancing up at me as though sizing me up. I wait quietly. Finally he barks, "Who sent you? Who told you to come here?"

I am thoroughly confused by both the tone and the question. I'm certain that Esther's primary care doctor explained who I am and the services that I might be able to offer, and that the family agreed to see me, so I can't understand why he's asking me this. I think for a minute before I reply.

"Nobody 'sent' me," I reply carefully, still smiling. "I was asked by Esther's doctors if I thought I might be able to help make Esther feel more comfortable, and so I volunteered to come by and see if I could offer any assistance in this area."

"No!" he cuts me off, now shouting at me. "I'll tell you who sent you. I fought vid the doctor here the other day, and they sent you to say that I'm crazy and unstable, to make everyone be against me."

Well, that explains it, I thought to myself. He has no idea who I am or what I do.

"I don't think I do what you think I do," I venture.

"You're from psychiatry! I know!"

I can't help chuckling. "No, no," I say. "I promise I'm not."

"So vhat are you?" he says, now fully locked on me.

I launch into my palliative care spiel—that my job is simply to add an additional layer of support, to help him and his wife think about difficult decisions they may have to make, to help manage Esther's symptoms, and generally to participate in her care by sometimes thinking outside the box.

He looks at me suspiciously. "Vhat, you know more than the intensive care doctors?" he says. "How can this be? The intensive care doctors know everything."

"Well," I say, "they know a lot of things I don't know, but there are a few things, like maybe helping relieve some of

Esther's symptoms, that I might know more about. I might have some unusual ideas about how we can do this."

"Ahhhh!" His face lights up, his eyes widen. "You're like the Google!"

I smile, surprised that this man who I assumed would never go near the Internet knows about search engines.

"Yes," I say. "I suppose you could put it that way. Regarding some aspects of medicine, you could say the palliative care team is like the Google."

"You know," he says, suddenly putting a hand on my arm and leaning in conspiratorially, "I don't even know what to put in the Google to find out about my daughter." There is a hint of sadness in his tone.

I'm moved by this man's slightly off-base perception of the Internet and its capabilities, by his implicit admission of helplessness, by his difficulty in even fully understanding what is wrong with his child. Even this new god, the Google, can't provide the answers he is seeking. The man who a moment ago was so hostile is now just a father, a supplicant looking for the right ritual, the right protocol, to give him answers about his child's illness and to help him find a way to make her better.

There is a long silence and I think to myself that maybe this is enough of an achievement for today. I can return tomorrow to continue slowly building trust. I'm about to excuse myself when he looks at my name tag.

"Valdman," he says. "A Yiddishe name."

"Yes." I smile, a bit uncomfortably. I'm not totally at ease with leveraging my religion and cultural identity for an "in" with this father, though I tell myself it's for the good of the child.

He looks a bit closer at the tag. "And Elisha, vhat a name! A strong name! The *navi* Elisha!" he says, using the Hebrew term for the biblical prophet Elisha.

"You know, he was bald, too," I say, trying to impress him by poking fun at my baldness while simultaneously displaying my familiarity with an obscure biblical passage.

"Yes, yes. I know the story. But more important, he vas a healer. A strong healer. He raised a boy from the dead. It's a good name for you."

We're quiet for a moment.

"You know the other story also?" he asks.

"Which one?"

"Vhat happens after the children call the *navi* Baldy."

I nod, knowing where this is heading.

"The children call Elisha 'Baldy,'" he goes on, "and he gets angry and he curses them, and then bears come and attack the children and kill them."

"I know," I say, "it's a terrible story. I prefer the one about Elisha raising the boy from the dead." I am very aware of his child, sedated and on life support, in the bed next to us.

"No!" He is excited again, emphatic. "It's a good story! A great story! It vasn't wrong. Everything is for a reason, everything is from there." He gestures up to heaven. "Sometimes it's raising the dead and sometimes it's God sending the bears, but it's all part of the same story. The trick is just to know when you're supposed to try to raise the dead and vhen you're supposed to let the bears come."

We sit there in silence for a few minutes, and then I get up, give him a pat on the shoulder, and tell him I'll come back tomorrow.

Acknowledgments

There are many people who, perhaps without their knowing it, helped me write this book. First and foremost, I need to thank the countless children and families who have allowed me to be a part of their care over the years. I have learned so much from each and every interaction, and I only hope that I have met their trust with respect and honor.

Much thanks to all of my colleagues and mentors, who supported and taught me through all of the challenges that make up a life in medicine. I particularly owe thanks to Lenny Wexler, who, in addition to remaining a friend and mentor throughout the many years since we first met, was also responsible for introducing me to his old colleague Mickey Weintraub at Hadassah, an introduction that changed my life.

Thank you to my colleagues in the world of palliative care, who welcomed me into the tribe and have continued to sustain me. I especially want to thank the entire PACT (Pediatric Advanced Care Team) at Boston Children's Hospital for putting the effort into helping reshape my career. Special thanks to Joanne Wolfe, who has been a mentor and a friend since day one, and who remains my go-to person—thanks for sticking with me!

My team at Columbia—Jen, Rosanna, and Chris—who listened to my musings and helped shape my thinking about palliative care as I wrote this book: I learned so much from working with you all.

To the staff of the Pediatric Hematology-Oncology Department at Hadassah: you welcomed me in and made me feel like family. You are a remarkable group, providing amazing, essential care in the face of a situation that can often only be described as surreal. No matter where I go, I will always consider you my family. I particularly want to thank Chana and Natan, who as chief nurses of the inpatient ward taught me so much and also gave me their friendship and support.

Fatma and Mickey—there are no words. You have been like a mother and father, sister and brother all in one. I will never again have colleagues with whom I feel so close and whom I value in the same way. I love you both.

While I was working on this book, a series of tragic and disturbing events unfolded at Hadassah, leading to the departure of all the pediatric oncologists on staff. Whether a department can be rebuilt remains to be seen. But what is certain is that it will be impossible to re-create quite the same special, beautiful world on the fifth floor that had been maintained and led by my colleagues and Mickey. Its absence will surely be felt by many, on both sides of the Green Line.

Thank you to my friends who made the years in Tel Aviv among the best, and certainly most fun, of my life. Josh, you've been like a brother; it wouldn't have been the same without you.

Altie Karper, who just happened to read an essay I wrote and decided to reach out to me in the email that ultimately led to this book: Thank you for taking a chance on me, for your patience, hard work, and diligent editing. It goes without saying that this book would not exist without you.

My family, to whom I owe everything: Eema and Abba, I am so grateful for everything you have given me over the years. This book would never have been possible without you. Adir and Merav, and now Tamara, Nevo, Yahav, Didi, and Shalev, you have always been there for me, and I can never truly thank you enough.

Finally, Sasha and Lev: Sasha, you believed in me and this project from the very start, even when I myself wasn't so sure. Thank you for taking a chance on me and supporting me through it all! And Lev, who has changed everything. Wherever you guys are, that's where home is.

ABOUT THE AUTHOR

Elisha Waldman is associate chief, division of pediatric palliative care, at the Ann and Robert H. Lurie Children's Hospital of Chicago. He was formerly medical director of pediatric palliative care at the Morgan Stanley Children's Hospital at Columbia University Medical Center in New York. He received his BA from Yale University and his medical degree from the Sackler School of Medicine in Tel Aviv. He also trained at Mount Sinai Medical Center and Memorial Sloan Kettering Cancer Center in New York, and at Boston Children's Hospital. His writing has appeared in *Bellevue Literary Review, The Hill, The Washington Post, The New York Times,* and *Time.* He lives in Chicago.